I don't know Katie, but I feel as if ⟨...⟩
other women whose hearts have ⟨...⟩
*Remembers the Barren* is precise⟨...⟩
have and what every pastor should read if he wants to be able to ⟨coun-⟩
members who are going through the pain of not being able to conceive
or of having repeated miscarriages.

**Rebecca Mayes**
**Wife and Mother**

*He Remembers the Barren* by Katie Schuermann is a gift. It is a gift for
men and women who cry and hope and pray for children. It is a gift for
mothers and fathers who don't know how to care for those who aren't.
Thank you, Katie, for helping me understand what to say and how to pray
for those who are barren. Most of all, thank you for pointing always to
our Lord, Jesus Christ, who never forgets His own and whose grace is
sufficient for us all.

**Deaconess Rose E. Adle**
**LCMS Board for International Mission**

With *He Remembers the Barren,* Katie Schuermann has penned
a significant devotional writing on a sensitive and emotional
subject. What is so beautiful about this book is how she deals with
childlessness in a Christ-centered and grace-full way, avoiding apathetic
fatalism on the one hand and self-pity on the other. The hymn
selections and prayers that conclude each chapter are pitch perfect. The
chapters are sensitive and compassionate without being emotionally
manipulative. This is a valuable resource for anyone who is having
difficulty conceiving or knows someone who is. As a pastor, I will be
sure to have a few copies available to give away.

**Rev. William M. Cwirla, Pastor**
**Holy Trinity Lutheran Church**
**Hacienda Heights, CA**

In *He Remembers the Barren,* Katie Schuermann tackles the difficult
subject of childlessness, a topic upon which society—and even at times,
the church—has remained largely silent. Joining the pious ranks of
women such as Hannah, who mourned her barrenness before the Lord,
Katie answers the complex question, "Is there a place for barren women
who still want to use their innate feminine qualities to nurture those
around them?" The suffering woman longing to be a mother will be

comforted by Christ crucified on every page of this book, and His mercy will move the reader from helplessness to hopefulness. *He Remembers the Barren* points continually to the cross, providing both a keen insight into an oft unspoken reality for many women within the church as well as sound Scripture to comfort and encourage.

**Adriane Dorr, Managing Editor**
**The Lutheran Witness**

*He Remembers the Barren* is a unique and greatly needed work. Its uniqueness comes from the perspective of the author. She personally understands barrenness and she personally understands Jesus Christ and His grace as revealed in Holy Scripture. Katie Schuermann artfully brings these two perspectives together and offers to the church a writing that will touch the hearts of many with needed empathy that only someone who has been there can bring and with needed hope and peace that only Jesus Christ can bring. This resource will also be a powerful tool in the hands of pastors, helping them understand barrenness and helping them minister to those dealing with it.

**James I. Lamb, Executive Director**
**Lutherans for Life**

In *He Remembers the Barren*, Katie has shone the light of the Gospel into the confusing and shame-ridden world of infertility, where it is so very desperately needed. She has articulated the perplexing feelings and experiences of so many women that those blessed with healthy fertility rarely comprehend, much less address faithfully and Christologically. Katie identifies the very painful struggles of barren women and, rather than giving into the temptation to wallow in self-pity, brings the sweet comfort that only Christ and Him crucified can deliver.

**Sandra Ostapowich**

*He Remembers the Barren* fills a glaring void in pro-life resources by addressing the grief and suffering of those Christian women, and men, who are unable to have children. Katie has been able to give voice to a deeply personal and taboo subject so that we may all empathize with, and learn from, our sisters in Christ who face this situation.

**Edward Szeto**
**Special Projects Coordinator, Life Ministries**
**LCMS World Relief and Human Care**

"Rejoice, O barren one who does not bear; Break forth and cry aloud, you who are not in labor!" (Isaiah 54:1 and Galatians 4:27) Prophet and apostle speak words counter-intuitive to our most basic human impulse -- be fruitful and multiply. How can there be joy in barrenness? *He Remembers the Barren* shows us the way. With moving prose and through people of great pathos, Katie Schuermann takes us on a journey through sorrow and joy, as we mourn with Robin and Katherine and Carol and Gina, and their husbands, barren but not broken, as they come to terms with the loneliness of this barren reality in their lives, Christ going with them all the way. But Katie's story of barrenness is also a story of hope. Real, authentic, and lyrical, *He Remembers the Barren* speaks to our hearts and gives voice to the yearnings of our souls. As we journey with Katie and her barren ones, we journey with Christ and in Christ, as she shows us how, through Him, even in barrenness, there can be joy inside our tears. Like Jerusalem at Isaiah's time, we come to understand that, in Christ, there is fecundity in barrenness. Comfort is here for Christ's broken ones who long to be fulfilled with the gift of children. Katie delivers at every level, always with Christ, never too much, and with Melissa DeGroot offering prayers along the way.

**Arthur A. Just, Jr., Ph.D.**
**Concordia Theological Seminary**
**Professor of Exegetical Theology and**
**Director of Deaconess Studies**

*He Remembers the Barren* distinguishes itself from other books because it reminds the readers that we are God's children, first and foremost, and that we each have a unique vocation, one that may or may not include motherhood. Through words and emotions, Katie paints clear pictures of the realities of barrenness, the effects on spouses, the loss of childbearing, and the peace that only God can provide. This book is a great comfort to hurting women and those who love them.

**Kristi Leckband**
**Wife and Mother**

*He Remembers the Barren* is helpful for not only those who are barren but for those who suffer, period. The author brings comfort to all of us through the appropriate use of God's Word which is the ultimate healing source, giving the reader peace and urging all of us to continue to learn and grow together in Christ, our Savior.

**Adrienne Rasmussen**

As a writer as well as a patient who has struggled with secondary infertility, I wore two hats while reading Katie's book. The writer in me relished the lyrical, honest prose. The patient in me nodded inwardly with each new chapter, "Yes, yes, that is exactly where I've been, what I've felt." But beyond the excellent writing and the truth of the infertile experience is a hope that can only spring from Christian faith. Yes, Katie is honest about her experiences with infertility, but even more importantly, she is a voice of faith in a dry desert of despair. Even while Katie wrestled with this painful subject, Christ's cheering presence shone through. Infertility is a lonely road to travel, but with Katie's encouraging and hopeful words, sisters in Christ will know the true blessing of fellowship.

**Julie Stiegemeyer**
**Author**

# He Remembers the Barren

For my barren sisters in Christ who feel they have been forgotten

"... and the Lord remembered her."
1 Samuel 1:19

# HE REMEMBERS THE BARREN

## Katie Schuermann

with collects by
**Dcs. Melissa A. DeGroot**

Lutheran Legacy
Fort Wayne, IN

Published by Lutheran Legacy
Copyright © 2011 Katie Schuermann

Scripture quotations are from The Holy Bible, English Standard Version˙ (ESV˙), copyright © 2001 by Crossway, a publishing ministry of Good News Publishers. Used by permission. All rights reserved.

Lutheran Legacy is a 501(c)3 not-for-profit organization. For more information about Lutheran Legacy visit, www.LutheranLegacy.org.

ISBN-13: 978-1-61327-001-1
ISBN-10: 1-61372-001-1
Library of Congress Control Number: 2011934845

# Contents

# Foreword

Martin Luther complained of those who perceive in Christ Jesus a "sweet security" which is not the consolation of the Gospel. Such "sweet security" Luther says cannot stand in the face of a bad conscience, sin, and death. For these enemies only the certainty of Jesus' cross and resurrection will do. *He Remembers the Barren* does not offer syrupy sweet security content on filling human emptiness with platitudes brimming with optimism but unable to enliven the hope which does not disappoint. Katie Schuermann knows that the Christian life is lived under the cross where disappointments remain and unfulfilled dreams haunt. Specifically, Katie writes as a barren woman to other women whose yearning for a child remains unanswered.

Reading these pages, three themes emerge: lament, Christ, and vocation. In our therapeutic age, where churches are too often dominated with praise songs that ooze with the "sweet security" mocked by Luther, we have lost the genre of lament which characterizes many of the psalms. In the psalms of lament, the Lord provides us a vehicle to bring our deepest pains, our unanswered questions, and our doubts into the light of His face. Lutheran theologian Oswald Bayer suggests that the psalms of lament allow us to pray even while the wound is kept open. Lament embodies complaint in praise as we remember God's past mercies and look forward to a future and uninterrupted praise of the Triune God. What Bayer has expressed

7

with theological rigor and clarity, Katie now embodies in her discussion of prayer as lament.

This is a book about a particular kind of loss, childlessness. But it is about much more. It is about the Child of Mary who has brought to fulfillment all that was promised to the patriarchs and prophets. This is a book that is about Christ who alone is the source of our joy and hope, our life and peace. Katie does not hold out a Jesus who will fix the problem of barrenness but a Jesus whose favor for sinners reaches to the very depths of our being. As Katie so aptly puts it, fulfillment is found not in the womb but in Christ. Writing with tenderness and a realism shaped by the cross, Katie makes a lively use of the Gospel to draw her sisters away from the temptations to self-pity and despair to the sure and certain promises of the Son of God recorded in the Scriptures and proclaimed in sermon and sacrament. Only in Christ is there true contentment.

Finally this is a book about vocation. Katie writes as a Lutheran who knows that the Christian life is a matter of being before doing. Our identity is given us in the name of the Triune God washed into the fabric of our lives in Holy Baptism. Called by the Holy Spirit through the Gospel we are now children of the Father through faith in Christ. The life we now live, we live by faith in Him even as we are active in love for the neighbor. Parents have been given the calling of bearing and rearing children. Not all have that vocation but every Christian has a calling to a life of faith in Christ and love for the neighbors God locates in our lives. Katie speaks of how women who are not mothers are also called to nurture and care for children. It is in the context of vocation that Katie deals with troublesome temptations to seek the gift of children in ways that God has not given. Faith learns how to receive all things from the hands of a good and gracious Lord knowing that His purpose for us is always good even though hidden from our eyes.

Katie Schuermann has given a tremendous gift to the church in writing this book. *He Remembers the Barren* breathes the wisdom of the cross. It will instruct and comfort women who desire to conceive but cannot. I also believe that my brother pastors will find it a useful piece to use in pastoral care. The inclusion of hymn stanzas and wonderfully-crafted prayers by Deaconess Melissa DeGroo

enhance this already excellent volume. May the Lord have good use
of it!

John T. Pless
Assistant Professor of Pastoral Ministry &
Director of Field Education
Concordia Theological Seminary
Fort Wayne, Indiana

Second Sunday in Advent 2009

# Chapter 1

# Portrait of a Barren Woman

I can pick them out of almost any crowd. It is not that we all look alike, but we all look at children and mothers the same way: guarded, quiet, even wistful. We grow silent and avoid eye contact during conversations about pregnancy, hoping no one will ask us if we have any children of our own. The questions — and, worse, the silence — that inevitably follow are so awkward . . . and painful.

I must be easy to pick out of a crowd, too, for that is how I met Sara. She found me. I felt her eyes on me as I politely declined the pizza that was offered to me at the party. I know she was watching when I refilled my water, carefully avoiding any of the wine or sugared sodas. She listened attentively whenever someone asked me about my age, my job, and my family, and her eyes met mine when I said that I did not have any children.

It did not take long for us to confide in each other that night. She had been married for ten years, and I had been married for seven. She had been diagnosed with Polycystic Ovarian Syndrome several years before, and I had more recently been diagnosed with insulin resistance. We both followed strict diets and exercise regimens, and we both had been trying for years to get pregnant.

Every time I look at Sara, I see myself. Her eyes reflect the same battle scars. She knows what it is like to hope and plan and dream each month, only to end up suffering through a private funeral every time her period starts. Sara is beautiful, witty, and smart, yet she feels like a failure in a crowd of mothers. She can turn a blank canvas into a beautiful painting and play sonatas on a cello, but she cannot make her husband a father. She is ashamed of her body and uncertain where she belongs. She is a woman but not a mother, and she is confused.

Sara and I ask the same questions. Why can't I get pregnant? What am I doing wrong? Am I unworthy? Is God punishing me? We look in the mirror and focus on what we do not have, questioning our value in the eyes of our Creator. Like Rachel and Hannah in the Old Testament, we pray to God and hope that He will remember us, forgetting all the while that God already has remembered us in Christ.

Sisters, we can waste such precious time in this life staring into a mirror. We can study our flesh until we have our faults and flaws memorized, but we end up learning nothing and going nowhere. Instead, we wander aimlessly down a long, winding path of navel-gazing where even the best and strongest of navigators can get lost. When you spend the whole of your journey looking at yourself, you miss the road signs that clearly mark your way.

Are you a baptized child of God? Then, you have put on Christ[1], and your Savior is perfect and holy. When God looks at you, He sees the redemptive work of His Son, and there lies your worth. We must pull our gaze from ourselves and look to the cross. In Christ's suffering and glory, we will find the answers, though the questions we ask will be different.

## Reading

Who is like the LORD our God,
    who is seated on high,
        who looks far down on the heavens and the earth?
He raises the poor from the dust and lifts the needy from the ash heap,
    to make them sit with princes,
        with the princes of his people.
He gives the barren woman a home,

---

1. Galatians 3:27

making her the joyous mother of children.
Praise the LORD! *Psalm 113:5-9*

## Collect

Let us pray ... Almighty God, out of man's side You created woman so that they could bear much fruit. Because of their disobedience, sin was inherited to all mankind. But in Your fruitfulness — out of Christ's pierced side — You created Your Church. While holy and blameless, Your Church still suffers the pangs of sin. Comfort those who desire to have children and cannot. Calm their fears and send Your Holy Spirit to guide couples to know what You would have them do. Embrace them with Your Word, and remind the Church's barren women that You do remember them, through Your Son, our Savior, Jesus Christ, who lives and reigns with You now and forever. Amen.

## Hymn

I build on this foundation,
    That Jesus and His blood
Alone are my salvation,
    My true, eternal good.
Without Him all that pleases
    Is valueless on earth;
The gifts I have from Jesus
    Alone have priceless worth.[2]

---

2. Paul Gerhardt, "If God Himself Be for Me," tr. Richard Massie (*Lutheran Service Book*, 724), stanza 2.

# Chapter 2

# Do I Have Any Control?

Sara knows her body well — *really* well. She knows what herbs regulate her liver, what foods support ovulation, and what exercises increase fertility. She obeys the decrees of her gynecologist and submits to the advice of her pathologist. She has gathered knowledge and studied her body to the point that she knows exactly when she ovulates. Sara does everything right in the eyes of science, yet Sara has not been able to conceive.

Not one to give up, Sara makes more doctors' appointments, consults with other nutritionists, starts drinking filtered water out of special plastic bottles, and incorporates supposedly tried-and-true techniques into her sex life. She spends two weeks out of every month preparing her body for conception, turning down coffee dates with friends and forgoing choir practice. She meditates on the prize until intimacy with her husband becomes just a means to an end, no longer a blessed union. She changes and controls what she can, but still no baby.

Sara knows she must be missing something. Doctors explained conception to her as a simple equation: if the right things come together in the right environment, a baby can be made. Sara checks out fertility books from the library, reads health magazines, consults with naturopathic physicians, and, like an addict seeking the next high, she embraces the next fertility fad that promises her success and fills her with desperate hope. After all, as long as she can

15

hope — as long as there is something she can change and control — then she might not really be . . . barren.

That word in and of itself is so cold. It brings to mind images of bare, empty arms and pale, sad faces. Who can help but picture Old Testament women with eyes that are wrinkled and heavy with shame? No woman in her right mind freely offers up such a descriptor of herself. "I have been married for ten years. I work for a marketing firm. I am barren." Talk about a conversation killer! No wonder Sara avoids such a label.

Looking up "barren" in the dictionary offers little consolation: *not productive; desolate; fruitless; lacking*. Sara has not produced a child. Sara feels desolate. Sara's womb is fruitless. Sara is lacking. Label or no, Sara is barren.

I am barren, too. I do not own a car seat, I have no maternity clothes to give away, and the only person I say prayers with at night is my husband. I have never been a mother, though I have pretended to be. As a child, I used to cradle my baby doll and change my Cabbage Patch Kid's clothes. I mothered — or smothered — my younger cousins every Thanksgiving and Christmas, picking them up and putting them down and holding their hands whether they wanted me to or not.

As an adult, I still pretend. I pick up my niece from school and play trucks with my nephew. I steal smiles from children at the grocery store, and I sit next to my pastor's children in church whenever he is busy preaching and his wife is playing the organ. One year, I even took out a subscription for the magazine, *Parenting*, telling myself that I was expanding my resources and knowledge base for teaching children's music classes. Who was I kidding?

The truth is that I am a woman, and I want to be a mother. Everything about me, from my anatomy to my marriage vows to my family tree, points me toward the vocation of motherhood. Why do I have a womb and breasts, if I am never to carry or suckle a child? If children are a blessing in marriage, then why is my quiver empty of arrows when so many unwed women are mothers twice and thrice over? Why am I not able to continue my family line and give birth to a child like my mother and her mother before? Frankly, it is confusing to be a woman but not a mother. No one knows what to do with me, including myself.

Such was the case when I sat next to Carol at a party. All of the women in the room were new to the area. We did not really know each other, so the conversation was light and meaningless. The hostess passed around markers and scraps of paper. "Write down a question and put it in this box. We'll pull out one question at a time and give everyone a chance to answer it."

Some of the questions were silly and fun. What's your favorite color? What celebrity do you think most looks like your husband? If you could go anywhere in the world, where would you go? All of us relaxed in each others' company. We nibbled on snacks and laughed at each others stories.

A woman across the room pulled the next question out of the box. "Do you want to have a child?" I felt my insides freeze. I tried to look nonchalant and hoped the woman to my left could not feel my heart racing. Had anyone noticed my face flush? A couple of younger women in the group began to talk about their plans to wait for a couple of years before trying to get pregnant. One was on the pill, and the other used a diaphragm. They listed off the reasons why it was good for them to wait: they needed to work to pay the bills; they wanted to have some time to practice just being married; they would be better stewards and more responsible parents if they waited until they had saved more money in the bank.

That is when I heard Carol gasp in some air. She had been holding her breath for too long. I saw the pools brimming in her eyes and the way her proud shoulders were starting to shake. She stood up to refill her drink in the kitchen, and I followed her. The sobs wracked her whole body up and down as she tried to recover her air. Her shoulders were defeated over the sink. I put my hands on her arms, not to comfort her, but to help her steady her breath.

"Why do we feel a need to control such things? Why do we think we even can?" she asked in between hiccups. "It makes me so sad." We looked at each other then, and we knew each other's sorrows and frustrations.

It was hard to walk back into that room of happy women. The party was too small for everyone not to have noticed our exit. The women would see my white face and Carol's red eyes and know our secret. Their smiles would be full of pity and their questions would be polite, but anything we could possibly say in response would be too much for them. It is always too much. No one really wants to know what it is like to be barren. Is that because, deep down, people really do think a woman can and should control her fertility? Or, is it because a barren woman challenges whether or not any of us really has any control?

Let's be honest. We all try to seek control where we feel we have none. A mother thinks that if she spends enough time talking with her son about alcohol, then he will not be tempted by it and can avoid the sin of drunkenness. While an honorable quest, the mother cannot really control her own son's sinful flesh in the end. A widow takes anti-depressants to take the edge off of the loss and loneliness she feels in her big, empty house during the day. The anti-depressants, however, cannot help her avoid the sting of pain that comes each morning when she awakes and remembers the one who is not there. A daughter glares at her mother and speaks sharply to her at the table, showing her displeasure in every way that she can. No matter what she says or does, however, the daughter cannot make her mother sign the permission slip for the senior class trip. A barren woman is no different. She seeks to control her body in every way, obeying the instructions of experts, hoping that she can make a baby.

Can a woman actually *control* her fertility and, therefore, her infertility? Medically speaking, a woman does have some control over her own physical body. There are, after all, often medical explanations for infertility, and a woman can make choices that directly affect her health and well-being. Maybe you know of someone who has been blessed to conceive a child after following the healing advice of a trusted doctor or after making a key change in her diet and exercise routine. In this physical, direct way, a woman has some influence in the situation. Yet, there are still those women who are unable to conceive, no matter how hard they try and in spite of what medicine they practice. In fact, even with the help of the most exact science offered by the world's top fertility specialists, as many as one-third of all the women seeking medical intervention for their

18

infertility never achieve a pregnancy.[1] If we do indeed have control, then why do these women never conceive?

The truth is that, in the end, we do not have ultimate control over our fertility. Scripture plainly tells us that God creates and sustains all living things.[2] We may attempt to understand and manipulate fertility science in an effort to achieve reproduction, but our own actions never alter the fact that we, as part of God's creation, are simply instruments in His act of procreation. Children are a heritage from the Lord[3] — a gift from Him — and that good gift is received, not manufactured or made. In His wisdom and in His time, God makes mothers of women. He has the hairs on our heads numbered, not to mention the eggs in our ovaries. Our gracious and loving God has control over our entire lives, not just our bodies.[4] All that happens to us in this life is according to His perfect will. Blessed be the name of the Lord.

## Reading

Unless the LORD builds the house,
    those who build it labor in vain.
Unless the LORD watches over the city,
    the watchman stays awake in vain.
It is in vain that you rise up early
    and go late to rest,
eating the bread of anxious toil;
    for he gives to his beloved sleep.
Behold, children are a heritage from the LORD,
    the fruit of the womb a reward. *Psalm 127:1-3*

---

1. "Ectopic Pregnancy & In Vitro Fertilization" with Dr. Kevin Voss, November 19, 2008

    http://www.issuesetc.org/podcast/Show103111908H1S1.mp3

2. Genesis 2:7; Psalm 36:6; Psalm 139:13-14; Hebrews 1:2-3; Colossians 1:17

3. Psalm 127:3

4. Matthew 10:29-31

## Collect

Let us pray . . . Lord, You give us a free will to govern ourselves in the temporal world, according to Your Word. Sometimes the choices set before us are not easy to make and can become idols to follow. Teach and guide us to live according to Your commands and rest in the freedom of the Gospel. You promise to give us peace, and in Christ, it is done. Remind us that You are in control and have authority over the eternal and temporal world. Thank You for always giving us what is good and redeeming in our lives through Jesus Christ our Savior. Amen.

## Hymn

God is my comfort and my trust,
    My hope and life abiding;
And to His counsel, wise and just,
    I yield, in Him confiding.
The very hairs, His Word declares,
    Upon my head He numbers.
By night and day God is my stay;
    He never sleeps nor slumbers.[5]

---

5. Albrecht von Preussen, "The Will of God Is Always Best," tr. *The Lutheran Hymnal*, 1941 (*Lutheran Service Book*, 758), stanza 2.

Chapter 3

# Why Am I Barren?

I take comfort in knowing God will make me a mother according to His perfect will and in His perfect time. I take comfort, that is, until I feel anew the emptiness in my arms and the heaviness in my heart. Within moments, my comfort turns to anger, and my faith turns to doubt. After all, if God gives the gift of children, then why am I still barren?

Sarai, Rachel, Hannah, Elizabeth . . . Scripture is filled with examples of women whose wombs were closed and opened by God. There are even accounts in the Old Testament where God causes entire villages or regions to be barren. We cannot ignore the fact that God has power to both bless and withhold His blessings from His people. We often turn to these accounts in our grief, trying to read into them a line of hope for our own barrenness. If God opened Hannah's womb, might He not open mine, as well? If I mourn and pray as she did, will God remember me, too? We spend so much time searching in Scripture for an answer to our own physical barrenness that we miss the point and, consequently, our true comfort.

In the Old Testament, barrenness carries with it a certain taboo. Barren women are shunned in their communities and scorned by other women for their childlessness. They cry out to the Lord for mercy and deliverance, yearning to be saved from a life of walking death. When God opens their wombs, they sing to the gracious Lord who has saved them. We see that barrenness in the Old Testament brings death, and fertility brings life and renewal — both given by a just, merciful God.

For Sarai and Rachel, however, barrenness has greater ramifications than just temporal death. The closing of their wombs means *eternal* death for all of us. As mothers in the Messianic line, their barrenness keeps Christ from coming into this world. In their stories, we find more than just the comfort of a God who gives barren women the gift of children. We find the comfort of a God who gives a barren, sinful world the gift of a Savior, Christ Jesus our Lord!

Through the wombs of Hannah and Elizabeth, God makes straight the way of the Savior of the world. Samuel, born of Hannah, grows up to anoint David, the great king of Israel from whose line the Messiah will come. John, born of Elizabeth, grows up to baptize Christ Himself, bearing witness to the Light of the World. By opening Hannah and Elizabeth's wombs, God clearly points the way to the Son of God that all might believe in Him.

After Jesus' birth in the New Testament, barrenness does not even seem to be an issue. In fact, few barren women are even mentioned. Is it because the barren woman is not important to God? No, it is because Christ has already come. Barrenness can no longer snuff out true Life, for death has been conquered by Christ's death and resurrection. Our lives are now made full in Christ Jesus, not in our own childbearing. Barrenness is now a non-issue — at least, it is a non-issue to our salvation. Yet, women still suffer on this earth in a barren state.

Why are there women who medically address their infertility and experience no healing — no success? Why are there women who are barren for no apparent reason? Oh, there may be medical explanations as to why the sperm is not meeting up with the egg, but there is no *reason* why one woman should be able to conceive over another. No reason, that is, except Sin.

I do not mean to suggest that a barren woman cannot conceive because of her own sin, or that she is enduring a special punishment for a sordid act she committed in her past. No, I am simply stating that there is suffering for everyone in this world *because* of Sin. God tells us in His Word that even one sin will separate us from Him,[1] and which of us is not guilty of that sentence? It started with Adam and Eve in the Garden of Eden,[2] and it continues with you and me today. We all — not just the barren — lie, gossip, covet, and hate our neighbors. We all put our hope and trust in things of this world — whether it be money, family, clothes, or fame — rather than in God. We are all guilty and stained before our Maker,[3] and we all need the redemption earned for us in Jesus' death and resurrection.[4]

The barren woman is not alone in her sinful state, so we cannot claim her barrenness to be a divine punishment for her sins. Does not the cancer patient suffer? What about the mother who loses her child? And the widow? Are these women being cosmically punished, as well? No, indeed! Praise be to God that He does not punish Christians for their sins! He does not need to; He already punished Christ in our place.

Why, then? Why am I barren? The truth is that we cannot know why. When sin entered the world, it was physical as well as spiritual. Some things happen to us today, like illnesses, ailments, and barrenness, that have nothing to do with us personally. It is just the reality of the fallen, messed-up world in which we live.

Yet, we do not despair. We are God's children, and we can eagerly anticipate His blessings in our lives.[5] We just do not know what those exact blessings will be or what form they will take. God gives the gift of children, but He gives other gifts, too.

Dear Sister, be assured of this: Whatever happens in your life, God will work it for your eternal good.[6] We know in Christ that God is merciful, and we know in His Word that He provides and cares for your every need.[7]

---

1. Isaiah 59:2; Ephesians 2:1; James 2:10
2. Romans 5:12, 19
3. Ecclesiastes 7:20; Matthew 15:19; James 4:17
4. John 3:16; Colossians 1:13-14
5. Psalm 103:13; Romans 8:32
6. Romans 8:28
7. Psalm 145:15-16

## Reading

The LORD is my chosen portion and my cup;
    You hold my lot.
The lines have fallen for me in pleasant places;
    indeed, I have a beautiful inheritance.
I bless the LORD who gives me counsel;
    in the night also my heart instructs me.
I have set the LORD always before me;
    because he is at my right hand, I shall not be shaken.
Therefore my heart is glad, and my whole being rejoices;
    my flesh also dwells secure.
For you will not abandon my soul to Sheol,
    or let your holy one see corruption.
You make known to me the path of life;
    in your presence there is fullness of joy;
At your right hand are pleasures forevermore. *Psalm 16:5-11*

## Collect

Let us pray ... Heavenly Father, You have given us our minds, bodies, and all our senses, our souls, and still preserve them even in the midst of a sinful world and flesh. You cared about all of these things enough that You sent Your perfect Son to take on flesh, suffer, and die so that we may have eternal life. Please be with the women who are at war with a body that will not bring forth children. Reassure them that Your grace sufficiently dwells within them by their baptism. Guide them to recognize their wholeness in Christ our Savior. Give them the peace You promise through our Lord, so they may serve You and be a bodily witness to Your mercy. In Jesus' name. Amen.

## Hymn

Well He knows what best to grant me;
    All the longing hopes that haunt me,
Joy and sorrow, have their day.
    I shall doubt His wisdom never;
As God wills, so be it ever;
    I commit to Him my way.[8]

---

8. *Andachtige Haus-Kirche,* "All Depends on Our Possessing," tr. Catherine Winkworth (*Lutheran Service Book,* 732), stanza 5.

# Chapter 4

# **Lord, to Whom Shall We Go?**

I get so angry sometimes.

One summer day, I stood in the middle of my kitchen with the phone clenched tightly in my fist. I had just learned that another good friend of mine was pregnant, bringing the count to a whopping total of nine. It was good news, really. My friend and her husband had been trying for years to conceive, and this was a cause for major celebration. I did not feel like celebrating, however. I felt like throwing the phone. Hard.

The shaking started in my shoulders and then crept down into my arms and legs. It was not long before my whole body was convulsing. Next, came the tears. They were silent and wet, sliding down my cheeks and falling unchecked onto my shirt front. I opened my mouth to release the wail building inside my chest, but no sound came out. I tried to breath, but the air seemed to hang suspended outside of my lungs, just out of reach.

I do not know how many moments I stood there frozen in time with no air, no comfort. I just remember feeling stifled and powerless, overwhelmed by the unfairness of the world. I wanted to scream, but even that power had been taken away from me. I felt helpless and out of control, and, like any injured animal backed into a corner, I got mad.

With a jerking motion, my lungs involuntarily pulled in a swoop of air. I coughed and spluttered as my lungs heaved in and out, trying to replace some of the oxygen that had been lost. It was then that I finally cried. It was not the high, shrilly cry of a child in fear. It was hoarse and guttural, like the whelp of a dog whose leg is caught in a trap.

In my despair and anger, I called on the name of my Lord. I cried out His name over and over again, not in praise and adoration, but in frustration and spite. *Really, Father? Is this the life you have for me?* I sank onto the floor in a pitiful pile, dropping the phone. I remember that it broke into pieces, the red battery spinning across the floor. I pounded my fists in my lap, rebelling like a child not getting her way. *So many blessings given to so many others, but what about me, Lord? What about me?!*

It felt so good to cry that day. Honestly, there was nothing else I could do. I had been dealt a bum hand of cards in life, and all my chips were spent. Other than wait for the game to be played out, all I could do was complain to the dealer. And, I did.

Maybe you can relate. Maybe you have been just as angry at God, shaking your fists at Him and gnashing your teeth. Maybe you have cried so hard that you have made yourself sick. Maybe you know the hopelessness, the frustration, and the anger that come with having no power to change your lot in life. Have you, too, sat empty and dejected on your kitchen floor, certain that God has passed over you in favor of others?

Then, good.

I do not mean to be flippant. I am not suggesting that it is good that you suffer. No, I am suggesting that it is good that you grieve in your suffering. It is good that you cry when you are in pain. It is good that you shout out in the darkness when you are confused and scared. It is good and healthy that you release the things you cannot control. Your barrenness is one way that creation groans in response to sin,[1] and it is unfair and painful and confusing. You are dealing with a death of sorts — with the loss of children you have never had — and you need to grieve.

Do not be afraid to call on the name of your Lord, even when it is in anger and spite. When you cry out to Him, at any time, you

---

1. Romans 8:22-23

are acknowledging His existence and His power. You are confessing Him as Lord. Your lamentation to God is the fruit of faith. We do not cry out to someone in whom we do not believe. It is in fear and doubt, the antithesis of faith, that we try to solve our own problems, carry our own burdens, and keep them hidden from God.

Lament to your Father in Heaven and tell Him you are angry, trusting that, in Christ, He will deal with you in mercy and love. After all, when we are busy shaking our fists at the sky, God is busy providing our daily bread. Does He not give us food, drink, clothing, shoes, house, home, and all that we need to support this body and life?

When we are certain God has turned His back on us, He steadfastly continues to come to us through His Word and in the Holy Supper.[2] Is He not present every Sunday in church where two or three are gathered in His name?[3] Is He not there when our pastor reads the Word and pronounces the forgiveness of sins?

Even though we turn our backs on God, He still turns His face toward us in His Son Jesus. "God shows His love for us in that while we were still sinners, Christ died for us."[4] No Heavenly Father could be more attentive, more present, nor more loving! Christ suffers with us, taking our barrenness upon His own shoulders on the cross, and sends us the Holy Spirit to give us the peace that surpasses all understanding. Where is God in the midst of our suffering? He is right here, offering us soothing balm for our wounds and taking on our suffering in our place. He is right where He promises to be, in His Word and Sacraments.

When we put on Christ in our baptism, God adopted us into His family.[5] We can now approach the throne of our Lord with confidence, as dear children approach their dear Father. He wants us to cast all of our cares upon Him,[6] even the unpleasant and unholy ones. Does not even the great King David vent his frustration and fear openly before God? David does not seem overly concerned that

2. Exodus 20:24b; John 1:1; Matthew 26:26-29
3. Matthew 18:20
4. Romans 5:8, ESV
5. Galatians 3:26-4:7
6. 1 Peter 5:7

his words will offend the Lord. Quite the contrary, David readily — even eagerly — shines a light on all of his ugly and fearful thoughts, confessing his sin and leaving nothing hidden before God. David's subsequent relief at his honest disclosures is apparent in the words of adoration and praise that quickly follow upon the heals of his lamentations.

Scripture even promises that when we do not have the words to tell God what we need, the Holy Spirit interprets our groaning for us before our Father in heaven.[7] In those wordless moments, we can also draw upon the church's rich heritage of prayer. In the Psalms, the great hymnbook of the Bible, God gives us His own words of lamentation, grief, and praise that we can speak back to Him. We can join our voice with the psalmist, calling upon the name of the Lord, trusting and knowing that God will hear and answer our prayers just as surely as He did those of King David. Even Christ on the cross turned to the words of a Psalm in His misery: "My God, My God, why have you forsaken me?"[8]

The great comfort in praying the Psalms is knowing that God's Word never returns void.[9] It accomplishes all that God intends. He hears our prayers and answers them,[10] and we are comforted. The next time you find yourself on the kitchen floor, call upon the name of the Lord. Know that when you join your voice with David in lamentation, just as surely, you will join with him again in singing a Psalm of praise.

## Reading

I waited patiently for the LORD;
    he inclined to me and heard my cry.
He drew me up from the pit of destruction,
    out of the miry bog,
and set my feet upon a rock,

---

7. Romans 8:26
8. Psalm 22:1a, ESV
9. Isaiah 55:10-11
10. Psalm 6:9; Proverbs 15:29; 1 Peter 3:12

making my steps secure.
He put a new song in my mouth,
    a song of praise to our God. *Psalm 40:1-3a*

## Collect

Let us pray . . . Heavenly Father, we do not cry out to You in unbelief. But, in anger, confusion, sadness, and affliction, we grieve for what we think we ought to have by Your good and gracious hand. We often miss that You are good and gracious. You, in fact, invite us to cry out to You. Our hurts are Your hurts in Christ Jesus. Just as Your Son hung upon the cross, crying out, "My God, my God, why have You forsaken me?" we, too, cry out in kind as sin, death, and Satan overwhelm us. Comfort us, Lord, to know that You have not forsaken us. May we, in Christ, continue by faith to grieve for that which You did not create and receive Your mercy and gifts of forgiveness, life, and salvation in Your Holy Word and Sacraments. Amen.

## Hymn

What God ordains is always good:
    Though I the cup am drinking
Which savors now of bitterness,
    I take it without shrinking.
      For after grief
      God gives relief,
My heart with comfort filling
And all my sorrow stilling.[11]

---

11. Samuel Rodigast, "What God Ordains Is Always Good," tr. *The Lutheran Hymnal,* 1941 (*Lutheran Service Book,* 760), stanza 5.

# Chapter 5

# How Long, O Lord, How Long?

"We expect to get pregnant," Janine told me one day. "No one tells us anything different."

Janine and Doug married straight out of college. They were happy, healthy, and eager to start their life together. It did not take long for them to desire children, as such a bounty seemed to be the natural fruit and blessing of their happy union.

"We were so excited," Janine remembered. "Friends of ours were getting pregnant the first month they tried, and we figured it would be the same for us. We fully expected to be holding our own baby by the end of the year."

One month, two months, three months . . . No pregnancy, but Janine tried to keep from feeling alarmed. Doug suggested that she go to a doctor to see if everything was okay, but Janine did not let herself even consider such a thing. Infertility, or whatever it was called, was not a part of her world. No one ever talked about it, and all of her friends seemed to be able to get pregnant right away. No, she was too young to have fertility problems. She would not panic. Instead, Janine plastered a smile on her face and closed the door tight against any feelings of doubt and fear.

Four months, five months . . . Time seemed to drag by in alternating states of confusion and frustration. Janine felt herself withdrawing from her friends. Whenever anyone at Bible study asked her about children, Janine answered that she and Doug were not really even trying yet to get pregnant. She was too embarrassed and frustrated to tell them the truth. Doug convinced her that it would not hurt anything to go to a doctor, so Janine made an appointment with a reproductive endocronologist.

"Yep, your cycle seems to be a little haywire," the doctor told her. "I am going to give you a prescription for Clomid. It should even things out. If you are not pregnant in a couple of months, give me a call." Janine felt relieved that the solution was so simple. She even began to feel a little bit excited. How foolish not to have gone to the doctor sooner!

Two months later, however, Janine called her doctor.

"Hmm . . . I'd like to do an ultrasound of your uterus, just to see if everything is okay. Let's also have your husband see a urologist for a semen analysis." The doctor still did not seem overly concerned about the situation, but Janine felt disappointed that the solution was not as simple as she had originally thought. A little seed of panic began to take root in her heart.

The ultrasound of Janine's uterus uncovered nothing abnormal, and the report from the urologist gave no offense. "Doug, you seem to have a low sperm count and low motility, but you should still be able to conceive with these numbers." A further ultrasound of Doug's testicles revealed a slightly enlarged varicocele. "This could affect the shape, speed, and number of your sperm, but I still see no cause for alarm. Janine, let's keep you on Clomid and see what happens."

One year, two years . . . Janine's life had become a steady flow of doctor's visits, medications, and tests. She sometimes felt ridiculous and embarrassed about it all, but mostly she just felt numb. What else could she do? Janine no longer tried to hide her fertility problems from her friends, but openly told her Bible study group about her and Doug's struggle to conceive. The outpouring of love that resulted comforted Janine a little, but she would much rather have had a baby than the sympathy of her friends.

The doctor ordered a hysterosalpingogram (HSG), an X-ray of the uterus and fallopian tubes. Janine found herself lying on a cold table in the hospital while ink was injected into her uterus. In an effort to quiet her anxiety and fear, Janine quitely sang "God Is

So Good" over and over again. The cold and discomfort would be worth it if this procedure actually revealed an answer to the infertility question.

"Everything looks great!" the technician exclaimed. Janine began to cry on the table, not from relief, but from frustration. Was there no answer? Was there nothing she could do to reverse her situation? Was she to be childess forever? "How long must I wait, O Lord, how long?" she cried.

Three years, four years . . . At the advice of another doctor, Janine began taking natural progesterone shots at the end of her cycle to help support a possible pregnancy. Time was ticking by, however, and still no baby had come. Janine began to feel desperate and helpless. She wanted to be a mother with all of her heart, yet nothing she and Doug did seemed to make a difference. An infertility specialist in the area ran a complete blood work test of Janine.

"You have Hashimoto's Thyroiditis, Janine," the specialist said. "Your immune system is attacking your thyroid gland, and that affects your metabolism which, in turn, can affect your fertility. I am going to prescribe a synthroid pill for you to take which will even out your levels." Janine was elated. Maybe this was the answer! Thank the Lord and sing His praise! She wanted to kiss the specialist and maybe even name her first child after him.

Yet, still no child came.

The specialist started Janine on injectable hormones in preparation for intrauterine insemination (IUI). For an entire month, Janine went on the birth control pill and injected herself with Lupron in an effort to regulate which hormones her body would release. The month after that, Janine began injecting specific hormones into her body in hopes of stimulating more than one egg follicle (preferably two or three) to mature at a time. Janine had her blood work checked every other day to know just how much hormone she should self-inject the following day. She also had a vaginal ultrasound to monitor the follicles.

Once the follicles were mature, Janine and Doug had a forty-hour window in which to submit a sperm donation and have that sperm injected into Janine's uterus with a long syringe. Before the injection, however, Doug's sperm were first put through a "wash" in which a centrifuge separated the bad sperm from the good sperm, causing the good to float to the top. Four to five days after the injection, Janine began taking progesterone pills to support a possible pregnancy.

The first time Janine started the injectible hormones, she could barely contain her hope. If ever she and Doug had a chance of conceiving, this was it! Science could not get much more exact than this. She went in for her daily blood work each day, happy and carefree. She did not even mind having a vaginal ultrasound. Yes, it was difficult to arrange her life around so many visits to the hospital, but it would all be worth it in the end.

Janine was standing in line at a store in the mall when a nurse from the hospital called her cell phone. "It looks like your body responded well to the hormones, Janine. Too well, in fact. You have six mature follicles at this time, and that is too many for us to safely continue with the procedure. The risk is too high for a multiple pregnancy. We'll have to start the process over again next month."

Janine clutched the Christmas presents she was waiting to purchase close to her chest. If she could just hold it together until she got to the car. "God is so good, God is so good..." she sang over and over again to herself. She paid for her purchases and fled to the parking lot. As soon as she shut her car door, the floodgates opened and her bitter disappointment poured out in cries of anguish. "How long, O Lord, how long?"

Five years, six years . . . Janine and Doug attempted two more IUI's after the first follicle debacle, yet Janine's period always came. She began to get angry at random strangers. The sight of mothers pushing strollers down the sidewalk became more than Janine could bear. She found herself avoiding the mall, so that she would not have to watch mothers younger than herself ride the carousel with their children.

The specialist recommended that Janine have laproscopic and hysteroscopic surgery to evaluate the condition of her uterus and fallopian tubes. The hysteroscopy revealed nothing new on the inside of her uterus, but the laproscopy revealed a spec of endometriosis on the edge of one fallopian tube, a fibroid on another, and a benign tumor in between one ovary and tube. The specialist re moved all of these and, in effect, also Janine's despair. Surely, this was what had been keeping them from getting pregnant up to this point! Janine and Doug eagerly performed another two-month IUI procedure, but they still did not get pregnant.

"Every time my period started, I would cry and cry," Janine confessed to me. "I remember rocking back and forth on my bed, singing 'God Is So Good' over and over and over again. It became my personal prayer, the words I would repeat to calm myself and try to make sense of the world. It all just seemed so unfair."

Janine wiped her eyes with a Kleenex. "People would constantly tell me to try this or that method to get pregnant. Some even said I was trying too hard! 'You just need to relax more,' they would say. I think people truly believed that I could control the situation, that there was something I personally could do to force a pregnancy. I felt such responsibility. Such failure. The pressure became almost more than I could bear."

Seven years, eight years . . . The specialist recommended that Janine and Doug try in vitro fertilization (IVF), but that was the one line they were not willing to cross. Having ethical issues with the procedure, Doug and Janine refused. "Well," the specialist said, "the only other thing I can suggest is that Doug work on his sperm's morphology."

"What else can we do?" Doug asked Janine, trying to bolster both of their spirits. Doug carefully maintained a healthy vitamin regimen, and he worked hard to lose more weight. Twenty pounds later, Doug's morphology was up to six percent, and he and Janine began gearing up for a fourth IUI. It was at this point that some adoption paperwork found its way onto Doug's desk at work.

"It was the strangest thing," Janine said. "After all the years of working to get pregnant — of being poked and scoped and injected — adoption just made sense. There was no dramatic scene or big conversion experience for us. It was the easiest thing to decide in our eight years of marriage. So, we dropped all of the fertility treatments and began the adoption process in earnest."

Janine picked up another Kleenex and began to weep softly. "Neither of us expected Grace. She is the great irony of our journey. After trying so hard and being told, 'No,' after so many years, we never expected to hear a, 'Yes,' from God. Yet, one day I missed my period, and there was little Grace inside of me."

Janine smiled through her tears as she remembered. "Neither of us believed it at first. We were both so unmindful of our fertility at that point, we almost did not trust the positive pregnancy test. It was such a miracle to hear her heartbeat. How it raced!"

Janine's face clouded over as quickly as the sun on a windy day. "But, God said, 'No' one more time. Grace died in my womb, and I have never felt such sadness." Janine took a minute to find her voice. "You know, I always desired to be pregnant, and God gave me that gift. Some women never even have that."

In the silence, I felt myself crying out in her stead, *How long, O Lord, how long?*

A tiny cry broke the silence. Janine's chin lifted and her eyes brightened to a sharp blue. She tilted her head in knowing anticipation. I almost gasped at the transformation. She reminded me of someone. She reminded me of my mother.

The tiny cry broke into a wail, floating into the living room from down the hall. "Excuse me," Janine smiled. She stood up and left the room. I heard the wail from down the hall change into a cry of delight.

Janine walked back into the room, bouncing a smiley, pudgy, baby boy. He squawked at me, causing Janine to laugh with delight. "I'd like you to meet my son, John."

My impulse was to reach out and squeeze that little bundle of blue and green with my own arms, but I resisted. The scene before me was too beautiful and perfect to interrupt. Janine positively glowed with confidence and contentment. She was calm, happy, and sure. A little red-eyed, yes, but the light that shone in her eyes was true and good. Little John was snuggling his mommy with all of his might, leaving a trail of drool on her brown shirt. It was clear to see that he did not want to be anywhere else than in his mommy's arms.

Janine's smile beamed across the room at me. "Doug and I adopted little John five months ago, and we have never been so happy. I am not pretending that our journey has been rosy and sweet, but we survived. We are stronger for it. I have a stronger trust in God and a stronger relationship with my husband because of it. I know with certainty that God is in control of my life and that he works all things for my good. I can now talk with women with whom I never would have been able to identify or understand before all of this. I also have John. Those are all very good gifts."

Janine laughed and kissed her baby boy. "God is so good!"

## Reading

Be gracious to me, O LORD, for I am languishing;
    heal me, O LORD, for my bones are troubled.
My soul also is greatly troubled.
    But you, O LORD — how long?
Turn, O LORD, deliver my life;
    save me for the sake of your steadfast love.
For in death there is no remembrance of you;
    in Sheol who will give you praise?
I am weary with my moaning;
    every night I flood my bed with tears;
    I drench my couch with my weeping.
My eye wastes away because of grief;
    it grows weak because of all my foes.
Depart from me, all you workers of evil,
    for the LORD has heard the sound of my weeping.
The LORD has heard my plea;
    the LORD accepts my prayer. *Psalm 6:2-9*

## Collect

Let us pray . . . Lord, in the midst of science and medical technology that You have ordained as good and helpful, let us be ever mindful that You still remain in authority over it. Give us the good sense to put our complete trust in You, regardless of medical outcomes, and award us the wisdom toward other opportunities. Just as we are Your adopted sons and daughters in Christ, put in our hearts a fervor to, "Let the little children come unto You," as You have charged. Whether You would have us adopt children or not,

may we constantly be led to understand that You are "so good."
In Jesus' name. Amen.

## Hymn

Lord, this I ask, O hear my plea,
    Deny me not this favor:
When Satan sorely troubles me,
    Then do not let me waver.
      O guard me well,
      My fear dispel,
Fulfill Your faithful saying:
    All who believe
    By grace receive
An answer to their praying.[1]

---

1. Albrecht von Preussen, "The Will of God Is Always Best," tr. *The Lutheran Hymnal,* 1941 (*Lutheran Service Book,* 758), stanza 3.

# Chapter 6

# How Far Is Too Far?

How many of us have spent entire seasons of our lives asking God, "Why can't I get pregnant?" We pray and seek and knock, hoping that the sheer fervor and sincerity of our pleas before God will influence a change. Yet, nothing happens, and, to add salt to the wound, our friends are getting pregnant all around us without even trying.

Why would a loving God withhold such blessings from us? Surely, the healer of the blind can open the wombs of believers. What is conception compared to the miracle of parting the Red Sea? God raised His friend Lazarus from the dead, so why would He hold out on us, His own children?

Certain that God is sitting indifferent on His throne, we turn away from Him like a defiant child and take matters into our own hands. We turn our back on His altar and, instead, bow down before the idol of fertility. We start visiting doctors whose ideals and ethics we know to be contrary to Scripture. We are back in the Garden of Eden, and the serpent is whispering in our ears: "Seek your own will. You know what is best." We begin to invest all of our energy, time, and resources into getting pregnant and, we hope, ultimately force the Creator's hand. We hold the fruit high and take a big, juicy bite.

Am I guilty of eating this fruit when I seek the help of an infertility doctor? No, healing medicine in and of itself is part of the daily bread God provides for us. Seeking medical attention where there is infirmity is natural and right. It is always appropriate to try to make the body whole. Some women require only a minor surgical procedure to remove a blockage from a fallopian tube before being able to conceive. Other women simply need shots of natural progesterone to raise their normally deficient hormone level in order to support a baby *in utero*. The technology available to us today is a gift from the Lord. It is part of how He richly and daily provides us with all that we need to support this body and life. Our sin comes in when we seek medical attention as a result of unbelief, when we no longer trust that God is good and gracious to us for Christ's sake.

God is our Creator, and we are His creation. We may want to have control over our bodies, but we will never truly have it. Each of our bodies is already engaged in a process of dying, and all women will eventually be infertile whether before or after menopause. The good news is that we do not have to be in control, because a good and gracious Lord who fearfully and wonderfully made us already is.

That devious, lying serpent! He would have us put our hope in conception, not in Jesus. He would have us focus on serving our own desires and needs rather than those of our neighbor. He would have us spend our money on expensive medical procedures rather than give it to the church. He would have us put our trust in our own desires and will rather than in the will of God. He would have us turn from life everlasting to eternal death.

What would God have us do? He would have us not despair. He would have our joy be complete in the fullness of Christ, not in conception. He would have us be released from the serpent's lie that contentment only comes through motherhood. God would have us receive His blessings and good gifts with open hearts and open hands, whatever those good gifts may be. Jesus said, "Peace I leave with you; My peace I give to you. Not as the world gives do I give to you. Let not your hearts be troubled, neither let them be afraid."[1]

Maybe it is best not to be so consumed with the question of whether or not to seek medical attention for infertility, but, rather,

---

1. John 14:27, ESV

ask ourselves *why* we seek medical attention. What motives influence your decision? Do you seek relief from an ailment that causes your health to suffer? Do you seek an answer to the puzzle that is your fertility? Do you desire closure after months, even years, of trying to get pregnant? These are all healthy motivations for seeking medical attention, because they simply seek a conclusion and physical relief. These motivations do not require a certain outcome of God, confusing the line between Creator and creation. Seeking medical attention for such reasons keeps you in a position to receive gifts from God, whatever those gifts may be.

Beware, though, the prowling serpent with his crafty, forked tongue. He wants you to have anything but the peace of God. He will try to convince you, just as he did Eve in the garden, that your will is best. He will encourage you to serve your own desires and wishes, even when it means trusting the words of your doctors over the words of your Creator. Do you wish to "make a baby" at the risk of hurting your neighbor? Do you think that having a baby is the only thing in life that can make you happy? Do you put your identity in motherhood rather than in your baptism? Will your faith in Jesus be upset if you do not conceive? Sisters, be wary of such emotional snares that would bind your faith to things temporal rather than to things eternal.

We live in an age of information and technology, and doctors have gathered valuable knowledge from years of researching the reproductive system. With knowledge, however, comes responsibility. The same medicine that can heal and support life can also be used to abuse — even abort — it.

For example, in vitro fertilization (IVF) appears to be healing medicine on the surface. However, upon closer inspection, the technology surrounding IVF pulls along a baggage train of ethical problems and complications. In the process of IVF, a woman's ovaries are hyper-stimulated by hormonal drugs to produce a surplus of matured eggs. A doctor then surgically removes, or "harvests," as many of the mature eggs as possible (often a dozen or more at one time) with a scope. These eggs are put in a petri dish and mixed with sperm from the male in hopes that they will fertilize and become embryos. Out of a dozen eggs, often as many as eight embryos result. The doctor will then typically replace two to four embryos back into the mother's uterus in hopes of implantation into the uteral lining. The remaining embryos in the petri dish are usually frozen to be used at a later time if the first implantation does not work.

In some cases, all embryos replaced in the woman's uterus implant and grow into fetuses. It is then that doctors can "selectively terminate" (or, destroy) one or more of the implanted fetuses in an effort to avoid the potential dangers that can accompany multiple births. The simple truth is that this act of termination is a breaking of the Fifth Commandment[2] of our Lord. We, as Christians, are commanded to neither hurt nor harm our neighbor in his body but help and support him in every physical need. This commandment includes children in our wombs.

There also still remain the frozen embryos. "Spare embryos, discarded embryos, embryos in storage, unwanted embryos" are all names you will hear tossed about in the medical community and media. We Christians give these embryos a more specific name: life. They are not simply byproducts of a medical procedure, available to be disposed of as any doctor or lobbyist sees fit. They are precious children, wanted and cherished by our Lord. The same benefits of life and salvation won for us by Christ on the cross were won for them, as well. Yet, the world sees the value and worth of these embryos being in death, not in life. The world would easily sacrifice the lives of these children for any advance that can be made in stem cell research. Sadly, many of the embryos will not even make it that far. Between twenty-five to fifty percent of frozen embryos typically die when thawed.[3] We cannot sit in ignorance of the death market that surrounds the lives of these children, nor can we ignore them.

Whatever sin and controversies may surround IVF, the children that are conceived and born to us through such procedures are still a heritage from the Lord. These children do not cease to be blessings and gifts from God simply because of the method by which they were conceived. We are not to think of these children as any-

---

2. Exodus 20:13

3. "Ectopic Pregnancy & In Vitro Fertilization" with Dr. Kevin Voss, November 19, 2008.
http://www.issuesetc.org/podcast/Show103111908H1S1.mp3

thing less than human beings who are wanted and cherished by our Lord. God's love is what makes any and every child valuable in this life, not the means of parentage. Whatever decisions and actions parents may regret, the children that result from such decisions and actions are to be celebrated as the precious treasures that they are.

It is the procedures surrounding IVF, not the children that result, that are in question. IVF procedures not only potentially break the Fifth Commandment, but they also confuse the one-flesh union between husband and wife. Since the egg and sperm are joined together outside of the body by a third party and later implanted in the womb, children can be "manufactured" outside of the one-flesh relationship. No longer are both (or even just) a husband and a wife required for procreation as God intended. This process takes us out of the mystery of procreation and into the realm of manufactured reproduction.

There are even more subtle ways in which the one-flesh union can also be undermined in reproductive science. Some doctors may ask your husband to masturbate in order to provide a semen sample for analysis. While the motivations behind seeking such medical attention may be healthy and sound, masturbation works against sexual intimacy between spouses. If your doctor asks you to do something that is potentially harmful to your marriage, ask him for an alternate method. In fact, if you have any questions about the ethics of a particular medical procedure or prescription, please do not hesitate to talk with your pastor. You may even have a pro-life doctor in your congregation or community with whom you can talk. Lutherans for Life, LCMS World Relief and Human Care, and the Concordia Bioethics Institute are three excellent organizations which help field such questions and direct us to Biblically-supported answers.

We sin when we make use of technologies that seek to transcend creation and our humanity. Attempting to control our bodies is actually a subtle form of idolatry. We break the First Commandment when we dethrone the True Creator in our hearts and replace Him with a make-shift god constructed of our own wishes and desires.

Maybe you have already made use of such technologies. Do you have regrets that steal your sleep and memories that plague your early morning hours? Do you suffer in private over choices you have made in the past? Remember, your help is in the name of the Lord, who made heaven and earth.[4] Christ, the Lamb of God, takes away the sin of the world. Confess your regrets to your pastor to receive the peace of absolution, and let it be done to you as you believe. "Repent therefore, and turn again, that your sins may be blotted out, that times of refreshing may come from the presence of the Lord."[5]

Now, Sister, in the words of Luther, "Go joyfully to your work, singing a hymn."[6]

## Reading

The LORD is merciful and gracious,
> slow to anger and abounding in steadfast love.
He will not always chide,
> nor will he keep his anger forever.
He does not deal with us according to our sins,
> nor repay us according to our iniquities.
For as high as the heavens are above the earth,
> so great is his steadfast love toward those who fear him;
As far as the east is from the west,
> so far does he remove our transgressions from us.
As a father shows compassion to his children,
> so the LORD shows compassion to those who fear him.
For he knows our frame;
> he remembers that we are dust.
As for man, his days are like grass;
> he flourishes like a flower of the field;
for the wind passes over it, and it is gone,
> and its place knows it no more.
But the steadfast love of the LORD is from everlasting to everlasting on those who fear him,
> and his righteousness to children's children,

---

4. Psalm 124:8

5. Acts 3:19-20a, ESV

6. Luther, Martin. *Luther's Small Catechism with Explanation*. St. Louis: Concordia Publishing House, 1986. 33.

to those who keep his covenant and remember to do his commandments. *Psalm 103: 8-18*

## Collect

Let us pray . . . Father, You created the Tree of Life in the garden.
When Your children fell into sin, we all were forbidden to eat from
its fruit. Yet, even so, we all still toil, trying to find it without You.
Father forgive us, for we still do not know what we do. Give us
the strength and faith to submit to Your will. Your timing. Your
gifts. Lead us to the other eternal Tree of Life that You provided,
the cross. The fruit of Jesus' suffering, death, and resurrection has
borne for us eternal life, salvation, and forgiveness of sins to all
who believe in Him. Help our unbelief in times of barren distress
and transgressions against You. Calm our fears and hold us close,
just as You have promised. In and through Jesus' name. Amen.

## Hymn

Oh, how blest it is to know:
 Were as scarlet my transgression,
It shall be as white as snow
 By Thy blood and bitter passion;
For these words I now believe:
 Jesus sinners doth receive. [7]

---

7. Erdmann Neumeister, "Jesus Sinners Doth Receive," tr. *The Lutheran
ymnal,* 1941 (*Lutheran Service Book,* 609), stanza 5.

# Chapter 7

## Do I Need to Be Fixed?

In a world which expects us to manage and control our fertility, it is natural for that same world to expect us to also manage and control our infertility. The pressure of the world's expectations pushed me right into the office of my pastor one day.

"Am I sinning when I don't look into my fertility problems?" I asked him point-blank.

"Why would you look into them?" he responded.

I studied the slope of the lawn outside the window. "To find answers, I guess."

"Do you need answers?"

I thought for a moment before shaking my head. "I have a peace about it all. Sometimes, though, I feel guilty after talking with people who think I should be seeking out more information. Some people tell me that I am not being a good steward of my body, that I should be trying harder to get pregnant while I am young."

Pastor leaned forward on his elbows and looked me in the eye. "There is nothing wrong with being at peace with God's will. That is one of God's good gifts to you. No one should try to make you grow discontented."

I met his gaze head-on. "Is it God's will for me to be barren?"

His voice was honest, yet kind. "Look around you. What does your life look like today? I don't know what God's will is for you tomorrow regarding motherhood, but He has not made you a mother today. It is good and right for you to be okay with that. I call that faith."

"Do people have a lack of faith, then, when they look into their fertility problems?"

Pastor took his time with his answer. "Some women need closure in this situation, and there is nothing wrong with them seeking answers to questions they may have about their personal health and fertility. It is also okay for them to employ healing medicine for any physical maladies they may discover. Healing medicine is another of God's good gifts to us. That being said, however, you are not sinning when you accept in good faith the quiver God has given you — whether it is full of arrows or not."

Pastor called my contentedness a gift from God that day, but many of my friends call it something else: inaction, resignation, carelessness, a symptom of denial. They love me and are concerned that I am unhealthy, both in the womb and in the head. They pick up my banner and wave it in my place, seeking solutions to the infertility riddle and trying to fix that which they see as broken.

Kelly picked up my banner one day after step aerobics class. "There are so many things you can do. We just need to find out what your body needs. Have you tried eating more cinnamon? It will help stabilize your blood sugar and keep your metabolism from interfering with ovulation."

She cornered me again at the grocery store the next week. "Stop at the herbalist on the corner of Jefferson and Cambridge on your way home. He has a special cocktail of herbs you should try. It is changing my cycle as we speak. I can literally feel my ovaries moving."

She leaned over her elliptical machine and panted to me the next day, "Are your prolactin levels high? You should check into that. I also think that maybe your progesterone levels are low at the end of your cycle."

I almost didn't answer the phone when I saw Kelly's name come up on the caller ID a few days later. "Has your period started, yet?" she asked.

That was too much. The line had been crossed, but I did not know how to tell her. I tried my best to adopt a joking tone of voice.

"Can we talk about something other than my uterus, Kelly? The rest of me is pretty interesting, too."

My hint must not have been strong enough. That evening, I received an email from Kelly inviting me to a chat session with a well-known authoress on fertility. "Just in case you want to ask her any questions," Kelly wrote.

I sat down with Kelly the next day at the gym and looked her straight in the eyes. "Kelly, I can tell that you care about me." Kelly nodded her head vigorously.

I cleared my throat. "I want to ask you a question. Do you think I need to be fixed?"

Kelly stared at me with blank eyes. "What do you mean?"

I tried to keep my gaze steady and calm. I could feel my own vulnerability start to steal the strength from my voice. "You have been asking me a lot of questions about my cycle and fertility. It seems that much of our time together is spent diagnosing my uterus. It makes me wonder if you are trying to fix me . . . if you are uncomfortable with the fact that I am barren."

"I just want to help," Kelly said.

My mind drifted back to the previous evening when I had first received Kelly's email invitation. I had felt so invaded and distressed. The thought of seeing Kelly again or even talking with her had left me feeling choked and anxious. I sat for a long time at the kitchen table, trying to shake off the feeling of dread that was weighing down my shoulders.

Why was I so afraid to see Kelly again? What could she possibly do or say that could offend me? After all, she really was just trying to help. I thought through my various conversations with Kelly and realized that, whatever her intentions, our interactions often left me feeling unworthy and disabled. Kelly seemed determined to find something in me to fix, and I was beginning to feel like my very life was coming up short.

In the dark stillness of that evening's vigil, a single idea came to light that helped me more than cinnamon or any herbalist's cocktail ever could: *I do not need to be fixed.*

Anxiety let loose its hold on my breath. Understanding teased the tension out of my shoulders while everything clicked into its proper place in my mind. I was afraid to see Kelly, because she treated me as a broken person in need of being fixed. Every conversation, every interaction, was propelled by her goal to change me into someone else — into a mother. In Kelly's eyes, I was not a whole person unless I conceived, and that both demeaned and exhausted me.

I thought back to my interactions with several other women during which I had felt the same stress and anxiety. Those women, too, had talked to me as though I was a sick patient on an examination table and they the wise diagnosticians. They wanted me to trust that their will for my life was best, ultimately bringing me to doubt the goodness of God's gifts for me today. It was so wearing to be seen — not as a woman with ideas and feelings and merit — but as a broken woman in need of being fixed.

Under the care of the Holy Spirit, my seed of epiphany gently flowered into a tender shoot of compassion. I saw in my mind's eye the faces of my dear friends who are also barren. Kelly's face flashed in front of me. I thought about her heart's desire to conceive a child. I reflected on her hard work, her tireless research and effort, to achieve the goal of a precious baby in the womb. I tried to see myself through her eyes, and I realized that my barrenness probably scared her. After all, if my barrenness cannot be fixed or reversed, then Kelly is faced with the reality that she, too, might also be "unfixable." Perhaps, in fact, her frequent attempts to fix me were actually vicarious attempts to fix herself.

Sitting across from my friend, I looked at her with shining eyes. My voice began to shake with honesty. "I am barren, Kelly. I am a healthy, strong, whole woman, yet I am barren. I do not know why I have never conceived a child. As far as my doctor can tell, both I and my husband are healthy individuals capable of conception. However, God in His wisdom, has never made us parents. We are trusting that God's will is already being done in our lives — yesterday, today, and tomorrow. We are content as we are. As my friend, I need to know that you can be content with me just as I am, too, barrenness and all."

Tears began to roll down Kelly's cheeks. I took her hand in mine. "I admire your knowledge of your own fertility, and I think it is good and right for you to be seeking knowledge and healing medi cine for your body. That is one of God's good gifts to us in this life, and, as your friend, I am here to listen to you and share in your joys and your sorrows. However, I do not need to be fixed of my barrenness in order to have value or to be a whole person. I was fixed in my baptism when I put on Christ. I am a whole woman, mother or not, in the eyes of my Creator. And, so are you."

Kelly could not look at me at this point. She let her eyes and nose run unchecked. I squeezed her hand and tried to lighten the mood a bit. "Don't worry, I have other parts of me that need fixing. Maybe we could get on those treadmills over there, and you could help me lose ten pounds off of my backside, instead?"

I am thankful for my pastor and the Gospel he preaches to me: I am baptized into Christ. My value is in my Savior, not in my womb. I do not need to be fixed of my barrenness to be content in this life, nor will being a mother make me more important in the eyes of my Heavenly Father. I still yearn to be a mother, but Christ's power is made perfect in my weakness and pain.[1] I am without child, but I am not without grace. And, His grace is sufficient for me. It is sufficient for you, too.

## Reading

The LORD is a stronghold for the oppressed,
    a stronghold in times of trouble.
And those who know your name put their trust in you,
    for you, O LORD, have not forsaken those who seek you.
Sing praises to the LORD, who sits enthroned in Zion!
    Tell among the peoples his deeds! *Psalm 9:9-11*

## Collect

Let us pray . . . Heavenly Father, You fixed us all at the cross two thousand years ago. In Christ, our sin was put to death. While we still experience the remnants of it in sickness, temporal punish-

---

1. 2 Corinthians 12:9-10

ment, death, and Satan's lures, our eternal home is secure. Our bodies, while ravaged with disease, are cloaked in Christ in our baptism. Because of Jesus we have peace and contentment. May we be ever comforted by this as our sinful natures sometimes cloud the eternal reality. Enable us to share this peace that passes all understanding with others. In Christ's name we pray. Amen.

## Hymn

The will of God is always best
    And shall be done forever;
And they who trust in Him are blest;
    He will forsake them never.
He helps indeed in time of need;
    He chastens with forbearing.
They who depend on God, their friend,
    Shall not be left despairing.[2]

---

2. Albrecht von Preussen, "The Will of God Is Always Best," tr. *The Lutheran Hymnal*, 1941 (*Lutheran Service Book*, 758), stanza 1.

# Chapter 8

## Why Does It Still Hurt?

There are some hurts that never really scar over. They remain open wounds that sting and fester. Sometimes, all it takes is one word from another person to make them start to bleed again.

Beth was having a really good day. She and her husband Jake had just moved from the country to the city two weeks before, and Beth had finally unpacked their last box. Everything was in its proper place, brownies were baking in the oven, and she and Jake were looking forward to the church party scheduled for later that evening. How exciting to get to know some new people!

Beth carried her platter of brownies into the parish hall and set them on the dessert table. She looked around nervously for a friendly face and was embarrassed to find that she was the first woman to arrive. Not knowing what else to do, she walked over to Jake and stood with the small cluster of men that had gathered in the doorway.

"Jake, this must be your bride," said a tall man with black glasses. He smiled and shook Beth's hand.

"Yes, this is my wife, Beth," Jake said, putting an arm around his wife. "Beth, this is Max Waverly. He is the vice president of the congregation."

"Hello," Beth said shyly.

"Pleased to meet you both," Max grinned. "Do you two have any children?"

Beth was ready for it. She had known this question would come up at the party, so she had carefully thought out her answer long before the brownies were even out of the oven. "No, we do not. We hope for them, though, should it be the Lord's will."

Max chuckled and clapped Jake on the shoulder. "Oh, now, I am afraid that poses quite a problem. You see, we have a church rule that you have to have children to stay members of this congregation. After all, we need to grow the church." He laughed at his own wit, oblivious to the pain he was inflicting. "Do you think you two could work on that?"

Before Beth could do anything about it, tears began to smart her eyes. She hastily pulled away from Jake's grip. "Excuse me, I think I left something out in the car."

Beth fled to the parking lot. "Get it together!" she said through clenched teeth, chastising herself for being so emotional. She had been just fine earlier that day, and she wanted so badly to make a good impression at their new church. Surely, she was not so weak as to let a stranger's comments get to her so fast! Yet, no matter how hard she fought it, Max's words crashed through all of her carefully constructed defenses until they tore at her open wound, causing it to bleed again.

My friend Sheila had a similar experience in church one day.

"There is a little boy named Zach who sits in front of me in church every week," Sheila confided. "He does everything he can to get me to smile during the service. He reaches for me with his chubby, little hands during the prayers, and he touches my arms when I stand and hold my hymnal." Sheila smiled as she recalled. "I always wait until after the service to pick him up, though."

One Sunday, as Sheila picked up Zach and gave him his weekly hug, a matron of the church came up and sadly patted Sheila's shoulder. "I bet you pretend every week that he is yours. Oh, dearie, you will have your turn someday." With a smile of pity, the matron turned around and walked away.

"I sit on the other side of the church, now," Sheila said with red eyes. "It is just easier to avoid Zach than to hear people say such things."

Amanda avoids people, too. Rather than be subjected to her extended family's ongoing commentary about her being the only adult grandchild not to have had any children yet, Amanda prefers to steer clear of family reunions. One day last summer, however, Amanda could not completely avoid her family at her grandmother's birthday party.

Cousin Don cornered her next to the deviled eggs. "When are you going to start having kids? You can't wait forever, you know." Amanda bit her tongue, reminding herself that Don was just oblivious to the fact that some people have difficulty conceiving.

Next to the sliced ham, Aunt Janice grabbed Amanda by the shoulders and kissed her cheek. "It is so good to see you, Mandy. Where is Jerry? Oh, he probably had to work." She sighed and shook her head. "I was hoping you would at least have had some little ones to bring home with you at this point, but it is what it is. Maybe you and Jerry will find time in your busy lives to work on your family, soon."

Amanda felt attacked by everyone's false assumptions and accusations, but she was careful not to let her guard down. She would not dissolve into tears in front of people who chose not to really know her. She felt some relief when she set her dinner plate down across the table from her grandmother.

"Happy Birthday, Grandma," Amanda said, smiling at the matriarch of her family.

Grandma looked up from her fried chicken and stared at Amanda. "It would be much happier if you would give me some great grandchildren."

We have all been in Beth, Sheila, and Amanda's shoes at one time or another. Many of us have fallen victim to similar drive-by comments made by parish members, coworkers, and even family. You would think that so much overexposure to the insensitivity of others would at least thicken our skins a bit and make us more resistant to pain. Yet, no matter how often we hear such hurtful remarks, they always seem to sting and burn. Sometimes, they even succeed in breaking us.

Most people have such good intentions. Our family and friends are just as confused and alarmed by our barrenness as we are, and their clumsy comments are usually an honest attempt to make sense of this unjust world. They think they are trying to comfort us, but, in truth, they are really giving voice to what comforts themselves. Barrenness does not seem such a scary foe to them if it can be labeled, defined, made trivial, or even ignored. We cannot so easily ignore our barrenness, however. The loss we experience at having no children stays with us every day. It becomes a part of who we are. Our daily interactions with others, our decisions and choices, our thoughts and dreams are directly affected by this thorn in our flesh. It twinges with our every move, reminding us it is there.

Some days are better than others. There may be entire seasons of our lives when we are so busy living and serving others that we are only aware of just a small irritation, something so trivial it can almost be forgotten. Yet, all it takes is one innocent comment from a stranger, the unexpected sight of a pregnant woman crossing the street, or the taunting whispers of Satan's minions to drive the thorn deeper into our flesh, turning our small irritation back into a gaping wound.

We may even come to a peace with the idea of never being a mother, but our thorn still causes us grief. Our heads can comprehend and cope with the reasons for our suffering, but our hearts still suffer from the pain. Some barren women think the thorn will go away entirely once they have children. We never really get rid of it, though. Even if we conceive and adopt, we still carry the painful scars of those empty years of wanting, waiting, and, in some cases, miscarrying. Those barren years are a fixed part of our histories. We can no more forget them than we can forget any other part of our identity in this life. Those memories stay with us, even upon the arrival of a newborn.

What are we to do, then? How are we to function in society with a wound that bleeds at the slightest provocation? Are we to resign ourselves to crumbling into embarrassing public outbursts of weeping every time a Max enters the picture? There is not much hope — or dignity — in a life like that. Are we to spend our days hiding from church matrons like Sheila and avoiding family functions like Amanda? That is both inconvenient and exhausting. What are we barren women to do?

We are to boast in our thorn.

Beth allowed herself two minutes to cry in the car before marching back into the parish hall. She knew that her red eyes would betray her weeping to everyone else in the room, but there was nothing she could do about that. These were definitely not the rosy circumstances under which she had imagined meeting new friends here at the church, but, then, her life had already turned out to be so different from what she had originally hoped and dreamed. Why should she pretend it to be anything different? God would give her strength to endure people's questions and comments, and she would be just fine. "Even if I cry again," Beth reminded herself, "My true friends will take me as I am, grief and all."

Sheila felt a small hand pull at her arm in the narthex after church one week. She looked down to find Zach grinning up at her. "See-la!" he said.

"He's been practicing your name all week," Zach's mom said proudly. "It was all I could do to keep him from yelling it out across the church during the sermon today. We miss you over there on the pulpit side."

Sheila bent down and picked up Zach. He wrapped his chubby arms around her neck and squeezed. "See-la! See-la!"

Sheila laughed and kissed Zach on the cheek for all of the church matrons in the world to see. Let them think what they wanted. Zach's opinion was the only one she was concerned about at the moment. "I have missed you, too, Zach. Be sure and save me a seat in church next week, okay?"

Amanda sighed and sat down across from her grandmother. It was time to say something, and Amanda knew it. "I want nothing more than to give you some great grandchildren, Grandma, but it's out of my control. Jerry and I have been trying for years, but it just hasn't happened. We are trying to be content with God's will and stay focused on the many, good gifts He has given us. It would help me out if you could focus on those good gifts, too. Sometimes, I feel very alone in this family." With that, Amanda buttered her roll and took a bite. "You do make the best rolls, Grammie."

Yes, we are to boast, not of our barrenness, but of the Lord whose power is made perfect in our weakness.[1] We run to wherever His Word is preached in its truth and purity, so that we might receive the words of eternal life and be comforted. We believe in His promises for our lives as revealed to us in His Word, and we look to Him for strength. We let our thorny flesh bleed, just like the Apostle Paul, knowing that Christ's power rests upon us, too. We keep living our lives in faith and let Jesus tend to our wounds.

What do we do when others scorn us with their words and pity us with their eyes? We boast of Christ's gifts of forgiveness and salvation won for us on the cross and given to us at the font.[2] We let others know that we are anything but pitiful in Christ. We ask our Savior to help us put the best construction on everything, so that we do not dwell on that which is evil and sinful. We petition Jesus to send us the Holy Spirit, so that we may return the ugliness and scorn of others with gentleness and kindness. We ask God to forgive all of us — the Maxes, the church matrons, our families, and ourselves — because we all say stupid things at one time or another. We pray to God for confidence in our barrenness because there is no shame in living a life under the cross.

We live in a sinful, fallen world, and our wounded flesh is always going to bleed. Our barrenness will always pain us to some degree and cause us grief. Yet, we are not left to suffer alone in this world. We do not live from day to day without hope for the future. Because of Christ's strength made perfect in our weakness, we can endure our thorn and press on towards the goal of eternal life in heaven where our barrenness will be turned into fruitfulness. Jesus, who was Himself crowned with many thorns, has already conquered sin, death, and the devil. Our thorn of barrenness is no match for Him, so go ahead and boast in Christ.

---

1. 2 Corinthians 12:9-10
2. Romans 6:3-5

## Reading

To you I lift up my eyes,
    O you who are enthroned in the heavens!
Behold, as the eyes of servants
    look to the hand of their master,
as the eyes of a maidservant
    to the hand of her mistress,
so our eyes look to the LORD our God,
    till he has mercy upon us.
Have mercy upon us, O LORD, have mercy upon us,
    for we have had more than enough of contempt.
Our soul has had more than enough
    of the scorn of those who are at ease,
    of the contempt of the proud. *Psalm 123*

## Collect

Let us pray . . . Lord, we live in a world that hates suffering. It cannot — or will not — believe that You are there when Your children are down and out, depressed, grieving, or in pain. Pain is the last thing it wants to associate with You. The world wants to think of You as someone other than who You really are. Even we, Your own children, struggle with this. Remind and comfort us that it was precisely through Your bitter sufferings and death that You delivered the world from sin in a blessed exchange at the cross. May all come to know that You abide with us always, in our joys and especially our sorrows. You know what we are feeling, have literally been to hell and back for us, and are with us now into eternity. Direct us, until our own temporal, dying breath, to receive You daily and much where You have always promised to be: in Your Word and Sacraments. In Your name we pray. Amen.

## Hymn

If thou but trust in God to guide thee
    And hope in Him through all thy ways,
He'll give thee strength, whate'er betide thee,

And bear thee through the evil days.
Who trusts in God's unchanging love
Builds on the rock that naught can move.[3]

---

3. Georg Neumark, "If Thou But Trust in God to Guide Thee," tr. Catherine Winkworth (*Lutheran Service Book*, 750), stanza 1.

# Chapter 9

# Will I Ever Be a Mother?

I remember when Mother's Day used to be a time of celebration. My father would let me and my sisters each pick out a gift for our mother. She would open them all at the breakfast table and smile warmly over each card. My mother seemed like royalty to me on that day. Being a mother must be a special, honorable thing, indeed, to have an entire day reserved just for her celebration.

This last Mother's Day, however, was the first time I felt left out of the celebration. I watched three generations of mothers greet each other warmly and proudly in the church pews. Men stood in the back of the nave, ready to hand out carnations to the honored parishioners. One grandmother wore a corsage her granddaughter had made just for her. It was a beautiful sight. I did not even think for a moment that I should not be joining in the celebration. That is, until an elderly mother being escorted into church by her adult daughter reached out and took my hand. "I guess I can't tell you 'Happy Mother's Day.' You are not a mother."

She meant it as an apology, but her words hit me like a punch to the gut. We were both embarrassed — she, because she had clumsily pointed out the obvious, and me, because I suddenly saw myself through her eyes. I was a childless, married woman. In a moment, I had somehow crossed a line that previously I had not known even existed. Never again would I be just an innocent daughter of the church, naturally joining in the celebration of the matriarchs around me. In the eyes of this woman and others, the daughter was gone and the non-mother — the woman without child — had stepped into her place. The shame that washed over me was instantaneous and paralyzing.

The grandmother with the home-made corsage overheard the awkward exchange and quickly came to my side. "She's not a mother, yet," the grandmother said with bright eyes, taking my arm. That grandmother sat by me — not her family — in church that day, and the love and compassion she extended to me that morning gave me a sense of value and self-worth when I felt I had neither. We all try to show each other grace in the best ways we can. I try to put the best construction on others' fumbling comments, and grandmothers try to give me hope.

I cannot help but wonder. Do I hope in vain? Will I ever be a mother? I know that God has given me the desire to be a mother. I also know that He has commanded me, via Adam and Eve in the garden, to be fruitful and multiply.[1] God's will for all mankind to have children is apparent, as He would not have given a command to His children that they could not carry out. Yet, sin entered the world, and our knowledge of evil began. So, here we are in a fallen world, barren and wondering what to do about it.

My friend Julie once said to me, "There is life-giving happening in your life even if it is not happening in your womb." Her words really struck me, and I found myself reflecting on them days after she said them. What life-giving is happening in my life?

I thought back to the hundreds of children I had cared for year after year in summer camps. I had definitely applied my share of Band-aids, braided dozens of heads, and comforted scores of homesick kids. I can still remember the lullabies I would sing to those sleepy little heads. Yes, I guess I had acted as a mother to those children and cared for their needs in the absence of their own mothers.

I thought about Irina, Lauren, Sam, Emily, Joe, and all of my music students over the years. I may not have taught them their first words nor helped them take their first steps, but I did teach them how to turn words into songs and how to use their feet to dance.

---

1. Genesis 1:27-28

opened my filing cabinet and pulled out the folder containing hand-drawn pictures and notes I had collected from students throughout my ten years of teaching. One picture in particular caught my attention. It was of a green, stick-figured lady with a too-large head and fingers as long as the arms. It was a picture of me, and I had never looked so beautiful. I remember the day Sam handed it to me and told me, "I love you, Miss Katie." Yes, I guess nurturing others' gifts and talents is a kind of mothering.

The faces of my nieces and nephews floated in front of me. I thought back to all of the times I had picked them up from school, fed them lunch, monitored their naps, and given them baths. I smiled to remember the honest confessions and secrets — those precious treasures — that my nieces and nephews felt could only be entrusted to me. "I told a lie, Aunt Katie." "I am scared, Aunt Katie." "I want to marry him, Aunt Katie." Yes, I guess I have even served as a mother confessor of sorts.

My mind drifted to the baptismal font. "From ancient times the Church has observed the custom of appointing sponsors for baptismal candidates and catechumens," Pastor read from the hymnal. "In the Evangelical Lutheran Church sponsors are to confess the faith expressed in the Apostles' Creed and taught in the Small Catechism. They are, whenever possible, to witness the Baptism of those they sponsor. They are to pray for them, support them in their ongoing instruction and nurture in the Christian faith, and encourage them toward the faithful reception of the Lord's Supper. They are at all times to be examples to them of the holy life of faith in Christ and love for the neighbor."

Pastor looked first at my husband and then at me. "Is it your intention to serve Lilian Cai as sponsors in the Christian faith?"

We answered as one. "Yes, with the help of God."

Pastor responded, "God enable you both to will and to do this faithful and loving work and with His grace fulfill what we are unable to do."

Amen. I looked down at little Lily and tried to wrap my mind around such a responsibility. Is there any other task assigned to a human being that is more important than instructing and encouraging a child in the Way? Is there a more honored — or more daunting — title a woman can hold than that of godmother? The spiritual rebirth of a child into God's family through water and Word is more precious even than that child's physical birth into this world through a woman's womb. Surely, this is an example of the "life-giving" of which my friend Julie spoke. God gives and sustains the life, and we promise to nurture it with prayer, instruction, and encouragement. God help us.

Godmother or not, every time we attend a baptism and join in with the congregation in saying "Amen," we are mothers. In that one word, we are both confessing faith in Jesus Christ to the baptismal candidate and promising to receive that child into our family in Jesus' name. We are no longer passive bystanders in that child's upbringing in the Faith but active participants. We instruct, encourage, protect, and defend the Faith into which that child has been brought. We are, in effect, spiritual mothers to every child in the church.

There are other ways in which we can mother those whom we have never birthed. God gives all of us the time and talent to physically and spiritually serve our little neighbors both in the church and the world. Some of you are Sunday school teachers, nurses, counselors, babysitters, and social workers. Others of you volunteer your sewing talents to make baptismal banners and quiet books for the lambs in the flock. Others, still, put on aprons and bake cookies every summer for Vacation Bible School. We are mistaken if we think we will not experience the blessings of family in this life, even in the absence of biological children.

Yet, there is still another way in which God can physically make us mothers, though it means letting go of some of our preconceived ideas of motherhood. Lorraine understood this perfectly well. She had been a widow for not quite two years when I first sat behind her in church. I admired her immediately. There was something about her countenance that seemed tried and true. Her hair was dusty white, her smile was steady, and her floral embroidered jacket did not quite fit over her stooped shoulders. The memories of her dead husband were still fresh in her mind and seemed always to be poised on the tip of her tongue.

"It will be two years next Tuesday," she whispered over her shoulder to me one Sunday before church started. I found myself trying to imagine a lifetime of learning to live with someone only to have to learn to live without him in the end. I reached out and put my hand on her shoulder.

We sat in silence for a few moments. Lorraine looked at me, then, and asked how long I had been married. "Five years," I said, and, without missing a beat, as if she could feel the breath that was caught in my throat, she said, "I used to cry every month. I wanted a child so badly. My sweet husband would comfort me and tell me that it was alright. That he was happy. We adopted, you know."

Adoption. It is not a new idea, yet it is one many of us do not consider every day. It is just not in our vocabulary. When we were young girls playing house, none of us ever thought to pretend to be mommies of adopted baby dolls. Our older sisters, aunts, and grandmothers did not model that behavior to most of us, nor did they equip us with such language. When you think about it, though, it is odd that the idea of adoption seems so foreign to us. We Christians, after all, already have personal experience with adoption. We have each been adopted into God's family. We know what it is like to be spiritually orphaned and without hope, wandering in the wilderness of sin and darkness. Only when God adopted us as his own children through Christ in Holy Baptism[2] did we begin to know the love and security of our safe, eternal home in the Church.

Do you and your husband desire to be parents? Do you both, in spite of your barrenness, still yearn to fill your house with children? Maybe it is time to prayerfully consider adopting a child. After all, you have love to give, and there are many orphaned children in need of a home such as yours. Just be mindful of the fact that children are still a heritage from the Lord, whether those children are birthed into our families or adopted into our homes. Children are God's gift to give, not ours to force. Pray about the idea, talk to your pastor, and share your thoughts and feelings with your family. If you find that life is presenting you with a green light, then open the door to the adoption process and trust that God will close it for you if it is

---

2. Galatians 3:26-4:7

not right. We can trust that when we petition, "Thy will be done," to our Father in Heaven, it will be done, indeed.

## Reading

Teach me your way, O LORD,
    that I may walk in your truth;
    unite my heart to fear your name.
I give thanks to you, O Lord my God, with my whole heart,
    and I will glorify your name forever.
For great is your steadfast love toward me;
    you have delivered my soul from the depths of Sheol.
*Psalm 86:11-13*

## Collect

Let us pray . . . Heavenly Father, You have ordained motherhood as a means by which to multiply Your creation. Motherhood is a blessing that many women physically experience. Be with and guide all women to know what You have given them in their vocations, whether they conceive or not. Remind us that You are steadfastly at work in all vocations to multiply Your kingdom. Thank You for the gift of children. Teach us what we are called to do through the care and raising of them in Your Church. Make us ever mindful to always point them to the cross and Your Word, that they may receive forgiveness of sins, eternal life, and salvation. In Jesus' Name. Amen.

## Hymn

Be patient and await His leisure
    In cheerful hope, with heart content
To take whate'er thy Father's pleasure
    And His discerning love hath sent,
Nor doubt our inmost wants are known
    To Him who chose us for His own.[3]

---

3. Georg Neumark, "If Thou But Trust in God to Guide Thee," tr. Catherin Winkworth (*Lutheran Service Book,* 750), stanza 3.

## Chapter 10

# What Are God's Good Gifts for Me?

God's good gifts often come to us in packages we do not expect.

My friend Mary is not barren. Quite the opposite, Mary is the mother of four beautiful saints, all under the age of five. She is amazing to watch. With the most serene expression on her face, Mary can cross a giant parking lot at a snail's pace with a baby carrier crooked in one elbow, a purse in the other, a diaper bag slung over a shoulder, and a toddling line of blue jeans and pigtails led by her free hand. She never complains about the number of diapers she changes in a day nor the length of time it takes her to buckle her kids into their car seats every time they need to take a drive.

In the world's eyes, Mary and I live opposite lives. From the books we read to the groceries we buy, Mary and I appear to be the antithesis of each other; however, upon closer inspection, we are the same. At least, our lives inspire the same kind of outspokenness in strangers.

One evening, Mary and I stood elbow-to-elbow at a reception. She was four months pregnant, and she had just switched over to wearing maternity clothes. She was vibrant and rosy-cheeked, radiant with the life thriving inside of her.

An elegant matron approached us and went right for Mary. "This must be your first child," she said with a knowing smile.

Mary returned the smile but shook her head, "No, this is actually my fourth."

The elegant woman's jaw dropped. "You look way too young to be having a fourth child! What is the age of your eldest?"

"He is not quite four." Mary gracefully kept her composure while the elegant woman lost her own.

"So close together!" the woman exclaimed. "Were you trying to have them that way?"

Mary replied, calmly, "We take them as the Lord gives them to us."

It was painful to watch my smart, talented friend be reduced to the status of a rabbit in the eyes of a stranger, so I tried to steer the conversation to an area that would help the elegant woman sputter a little less. "I really like your yellow shoes! Where did you get them?"

Mary had a chance to return the favor the following week. We both sat at the same table at a ladies' luncheon, enjoying the hot tea and each others' company. A red-haired woman sitting across the table looked at me over her glasses and asked point-blank, "Do you have any children?"

"No," I replied, cautiously hiding my face behind my cup.

"Why not? Are you on the pill?" The woman's eyes were bold and her tone accusing.

"No," I blushed, "I am not."

I saw Mary shift in her chair and take a sip of tea.

"Are you trying to get pregnant?" the woman dug a little further.

Mary leaned forward in her seat and engaged the red-haired woman directly. "Your hairstyle is adorable. Who cuts your hair?"

Mary and I have been friends for only three years, yet we have found each other to be steady allies in an unsteady world. We bolster each other up when others try to weigh us down with judgments for having too many or too few children. The fruit of our wombs is markedly different, but we find camaraderie in having the same respect for life and approach to fertility. We know that children are a heritage from the Lord, and we trust God to give them to us according to His will. We welcome pregnancies as they come or as they do not come. We pray the same prayer to the same God: "Thy will be done." Our results look so different, but our faith is the same.

Who could have predicted that a mother of four would know and understand me better than any other barren woman? Mary's friendship is definitely one of God's good gifts to me, and I am so thankful to have someone in my life who prays for me, loves me, and supports me regardless of my fertility status. It makes me wonder, though, just how many Marys have I turned away over the years with my own prejudices? On more than one occasion, I have shunned the friendships of other women simply because they happened to be mothers. I have judged them solely on their circumstances, just like the elegant woman did of Mary, and made assumptions about their lives before really knowing them, just like the red-haired woman did of me. I have let my own expectations and prejudices make me blind to the gifts of compassion God would provide for me in others.

Guard yourself against such entrapments. The truth is that many women in the body of Christ can empathize with your pain, even if their trials do not look exactly like your own. Some women conceive on their honeymoons, and they do not feel any joy or excitement about their pregnancies. They may even go so far as to regret the children in their wombs, feeling cheated out of much-desired careers and time with their husbands. These women suffer just as much pain as we do when confronted with circumstances they cannot control. They experience the same frustration and despair. Perhaps they even covet women who, like ourselves, are barren. We may carry different crosses in this life, but our knowledge of suffering and grief make us ready friends and empathetic supporters of each other.

Mary's friendship serves to remind me of the many other good gifts God gives to me on a daily basis. For example, God makes each of us stewards of gifts of time. As a mother, Mary's gift of time is regularly spent in service to her children. Meal times, nap times, school activities, and doctor's appointments regularly dictate the course of Mary's every day, and she serves her little neighbors in love and grace by caring for their daily needs. The gift of time of which God has made me a steward, however, does not require me to take care of children of my own. As a result, I am free to spend more time taking care of my family in Christ at large. I can pick up Mrs. Gardner on my way to Wednesday morning Bible study, because I do not need to monitor naps at home. I can serve lunch to the school children in the cafeteria, because I do not have anyone in need of being served lunch at home. I can attend the local Lutheran High School volleyball and football games in the afternoons to cheer on our youth, because I do not need to meet children at the bus stop after school. I can ring bells and sing in the choir during both the early and late church services, because I do not need to tend to youngsters in the pews. Overall, I have a flexibility of schedule which enables me to give more time in service to my church.

God makes each of us stewards of gifts of money, as well. As a mother, Mary's gift of money is often spent on new shoes, coats, and food for her growing children. She serves her family by paying for ball gloves and piano lessons, often sacrificing new clothes and hobbies for herself. The gift of money of which God has made me a steward, however, does not require me to fund the livelihood of children of my own. Instead, I am free to give money to support the livelihood of others in the church, such as making a monthly donation to support a seminary student or a missionary worker for LCMS World Mission. God asks each of us to serve our neighbor with the resources He has given us. Some of us just serve taller neighbors than others.

As a barren woman, I am in a unique position to give to the church in different ways — and sometimes in different quantities — than women who have children. True, maybe I would prefer to have my own children to care for like Mary, but God in His wisdom has given me different gifts to share and different neighbors to serve. God also very clearly instructs me in the Ninth and Tenth Commandments[1] not to covet who Mary is and what she has but, instead, to help and be of service to her in keeping that which is hers.

God's law is so wise. It knows that navel-gazing will most certainly lead me to despair. It tries to protect me from becoming a green-eyed monster by commanding me to serve my neighbor instead of myself. It tries to curb my behavior away from self-pity and jealousy and, instead, redirect it towards contentment in life and

---

1. Exodus 20:17

service of others.[2] It tries to keep me from sin and the death it inevitably brings. However, the same law which tries to protect also convicts me, for I am already guilty. I have not only coveted my neighbor's children, but I have failed her in keeping and preserving them. I have sinned and fallen short of the glory of God.

Praise God that Jesus offered Himself as a ransom for my sin! I can rest in the peace of knowing that the absolution spoken by my pastor in the stead of Christ is spoken for my sake. I can remember my baptism and rejoice that God has marked me as His own through water and the Word. I am redeemed by the blood of the Lamb, and He beckons me to the table to be refreshed and strengthened in my faith through the eating of His Body and the drinking of His Blood. I am forgiven of my sins, and I will be raised in my flesh on the last day to behold my Savior with my own eyes. Honestly, I can think of no better gift than that.

## Reading

The law of the LORD is perfect,
    reviving the soul;
the testimony of the LORD is sure,
    making wise the simple;
the precepts of the LORD are right,
    rejoicing the heart;
the commandment of the LORD is pure,
    enlightening the eyes;
the fear of the LORD is clean,
    enduring forever;
the rules of the LORD are true,
    and righteous altogether.
More to be desired are they than gold,
    even much fine gold;
    sweeter also than honey and drippings of the honeycomb.
Moreover, by them is your servant warned;
    in keeping them there is great reward.
Who can discern his errors?

---

2. Luke 10:27

Declare me innocent from hidden faults.
Keep back your servant also from presumptuous sins;
    let them not have dominion over me!
Then shall I be blameless,
    and innocent of great transgression.
Let the words of my mouth and the meditation of my heart
    be acceptable in your sight,
O LORD, my rock and my redeemer. *Psalm 19:7-14*

## Collect

Let us pray . . . Heavenly Father, You want to give us every gift imaginable. This includes earthly gifts, such as house, family, food, clothing, and all we physically and emotionally need to support our bodies in this life. You also give us what we need to live eternally: Your Son. Jesus binds Himself with us, even now, as often as we eat and drink His Body and Blood in the Lord's Supper, in the daily remembrance of our baptism, and in the Word — who is truly our Lord, as well — so that we might be with You. All these things we receive both without any merit or worthiness in us, but because You are holy, gracious, and good. You are the true Gift-Giver to all the world. Thank You for all Your gifts, both earthly and heavenly. In Christ's name. Amen.

## Hymn

By grace! None dare lay claim to merit;
    Our works and conduct have no worth.
God in His love sent our Redeemer,
    Christ Jesus, to this sinful earth;
His death did for our sins atone,
    And we are saved by grace alone.[3]

---

3. Christian Ludwig Scheidt, "By Grace I'm Saved," tr. *The Lutheran Hymnal*, 1941 (*Lutheran Service Book,* 566), stanza 2.

# Chapter 11

# In Sickness and in Health?

When a man leaves his father and mother and holds fast to his wife, they become one flesh.[1] According to God's perfect design, children are the natural fruit of this blessed, one-flesh union. The unnatural state of barrenness, therefore, is not a burden for the wife to bear alone. A husband and wife are barren *together*.

This is not an invitation for you to immediately turn on your husband, to start poking and prodding him in a frenzy to find out if his genetics are contributing to your barren state. Ultimately, it does not really matter if physical barrenness comes from your womb or his sperm. You are one flesh, and you each suffer together from barrenness regardless of the exact medical diagnosis. Rather than thinking of your husband as a lab rat, consider the fact that he is a man who has vowed to love you in good times and in bad, in sickness and in health, for better or for worse. He is your built-in supporter, your fierce protector, and your greatest advocate. He is one of God's greatest gifts to you in this life.

Have you stopped to consider the fact that your husband understands the pain and suffering that come with barrenness? You share the same home, so your husband knows exactly what it is like to pass by the spare bedroom and wonder if it will ever be turned into a nursery. He, too, is painfully aware of the fact that family dinner and prayer times are attended by only two people. You share the

1. Genesis 2:24

same family as your husband, so he gets teased by aunts and uncles every Christmas like you. He is just as angered by the injustice of how easily and frequently your unwed cousins get pregnant. You also attend the same dinner parties, so your husband fields fertility questions and wisecracks from the same oblivious strangers as you. More than that, he sees the way those questions and comments cause you, his bride, to suffer.

You do not have to carry the burden of barrenness alone but have the support of a man who has committed to love you as Christ loves the church. Do you ever ask this man for help? Do you confess to him your fears and doubts? Does he know how guilty you feel for not being able to bear him children? Do you let him see you weep? Sometimes, the very comfort you crave can be found lying on the pillow next to you.

The same is true for your husband. You are one of God's good gifts to him in this life. Woman was made from man's rib that he might have a helpmate and companion to share his days. Your husband is hurting, too, even if he does not tell you about his suffering. The absence of children is an attack on his identity, his manhood, and his dream for continuing his family line. Do you pray for him, take care of his daily needs, and nurture his emotional and physical health? Do you work hard to make his home a place of refuge and rest from the world's stresses? Do you spend your days tending to his needs or simply drawing attention to your own?

Your one-flesh union is intended to be a source of comfort and support for both of you, a safe zone where unconditional love and forgiveness abound. However, marriage can just as easily become a minefield ridden with accusations and blame, especially when it carries the stress and burden of barrenness on its shoulders. Such was the case for Katherine and Paul.

Katherine was so mad. Her period had started two days earlier and Paul acted as if nothing was wrong. He just went about his day making calls for work and taking the dog for walks. He never once asked her how she was doing or even acknowledged that anything had happened. It was all Katherine could do to keep from throwing her cup of hot tea on Paul when he picked up a book to read that night.

"How can you sit there and pretend like nothing is wrong?" Katherine fumed.

Paul kept reading.

"Are you just going to ignore me the whole evening?" Katherine's voice dripped with venom.

"I am not ignoring you." Paul's eyes never left the page. "I am reading a book."

Katherine felt hot tears sear her cheeks. "I am bleeding, and all you want to do is read a book?"

Paul sighed. "I am just really tired, Kathy. It has been a long month, and I need a break."

"A break from what?" Katherine cried. "From your wife?"

"No," Paul said quietly, shutting his book. "A break from all of the drama."

Katherine bit her lip and shook her head. "I can't believe you just said that."

Paul ran his hand through his hair. "What am I supposed to say?"

"Well, you could start with, 'How are you? Is there anything I can do for you? Are you in any pain?'" Katherine's voice cracked with emotion.

Paul rubbed his eyes. "Kathy, I never know what to say to you. When you are stressed, I never seem to be able to say anything right."

"When *I* am stressed?" Kathy's eyes flashed. "That's just it! We are not pregnant, and *I* am the only one who is stressed. You don't seem to care if we have a baby or not. I am alone in this," Kathy sobbed into her hands.

Paul sighed again and shook his head. He sat still for a few moments, staring at the floor. Suddenly, he stood up and grabbed his jacket. "I'm going to take the dog for a walk."

Katherine looked up and watched as Paul stood with his back to her, shrugging his shoulders into his jacket. She choked back a sob and ran down the hall, slamming the bedroom door behind her.

There are so many times when I, like Katherine, am blinded by my own emotions. I pick fights with my husband in an effort to get him to notice me. I ask him questions but do not really listen to his answers. I focus on my own needs, taking whatever he says and twisting his words to serve my own agenda. I project my expectations of life on him, condemning him in my heart when he does not react to a situation just as I think he should. I turn from loving and serving him to loving and serving myself.

It never works, though. I never leave such arguments feeling satisfied and happy. Instead, like Katherine, I usually run off to a closed room to lick my wounds and wallow in self pity. I spend the next hour making mental lists of all of the reasons I am right and my husband is wrong, building up a fortress of self-righteousness to stave off the winds of conviction the Holy Spirit inevitably blows my way. My fortress never stands for very long, however. God always finds the weak spots in my stronghold, and, more often than not, He uses my husband to bring it crashing down.

Katherine lay face down on the bed, sobbing into her pillow. She heard Paul's footsteps follow her down the hall. The door opened and the bed creaked as he sat down next to her.

"Kathy," Paul said quietly, "I am sorry."

Katherine stubbornly did not answer him.

Paul rested his hand on her back. "Honey, I have not been very good at talking with you, lately. I just don't know what to say. I am so tired and frustrated." He started rubbing her back, taking his time. "I do feel disappointed that we are not pregnant, but I didn't want to say anything. I was afraid it would make you more upset. I didn't want to make you feel any worse."

Katherine sniffed and wiped her face with her sleeve.

"I want to have a child more than anything," Paul continued, "But I am tired of being disappointed month after month. There just seems to be nothing I can do to change the situation. Sometimes I feel like I am going to snap." Paul's shoulders sagged in defeat. "I just wish there was something I could do."

Katherine's voice was quiet. "There is something you can do."

"What?" Paul asked, leaning closer to his wife.

"You can hold me."

Paul tenderly wrapped his arms around Katherine, pulling her onto his lap. Katherine buried her face in his neck. "I am sorry, too," she said. "I have been acting like a child."

"I haven't acted much better," Paul said into her hair.

"I feel so out of control," she said. "I just get so angry. And scared."

"Me, too," He said. "Me, too."

I wonder how many arguments could be avoided in barren marriages if we wives remembered one important truth: man is not woman. More directly, your husband is not you. Your husband may perfectly understand the circumstances of being childless, but he is not necessarily going to react to those circumstances the same as you. In fact, he is most likely going to think about and cope with those circumstances much differently, and that is healthy and just as it should be. You were not made by God to be the same.

If you wake up each morning with expectations of how your husband should think and feel, you might as well put on war paint instead of make-up. You will have to fight your husband to make him think and behave like yourself, and I am pretty sure you will be unhappy with the results in the end, anyway. Rather, let your husband have his own, honest reactions to the cross of barrenness that he bears. By watching him, listening to him, and loving him, you will better learn how to help shoulder his burden when he needs it.

It is also important to remember that your husband is not psychic. He cannot read your mind. He may not even know you well enough, yet, to pick up on all of your emotional triggers. Barrenness often comes to light within the first few years of marriage, and that is a time when a husband and wife are still learning how to be married, let alone how to be good at it. Even ten or twenty years into a marriage, a wife still cannot expect her husband to be able to predict what she needs all of the time. Instead, it is important that she *tell* him what she needs, so that he will have the opportunity to help and support her at the appropriate times.

A husband wants to be able to help his wife. He wants to take care of her and provide for her needs. He wants to put food on her table and clothes in her closet. He wants to be able to give her children. In barrenness, a husband not only feels the pain of not being a father, but he also feels the pain of not being able to provide for his wife. He is broken by the fact there is nothing he can do to control the situation.

Thankfully, your husband is not alone in his suffering. He has you. Together, you can shoulder each others burdens, because Christ first bore all of your burdens on the cross. You can pray for each other and with each other, knowing that where two or more are gathered in His name, there is Christ in the midst of you. You can begin and end the day together in God's Word, meditating on His promises for you, both in this life and in eternity. You can provide mutual consolation — even exhortation — when it is needed in the dark hours of the night, reading aloud the Psalms to chase away the demons at your pillows. You can kneel at the altar together and receive Christ's Body and Blood for the salvation of your souls and the refreshment of your spirits. You can remind each other that your marriage, instituted by God, is no less blessed nor incomplete because of barrenness. Your one-flesh union is good and right, even in the absence of children.

Most important of all, you can forgive each other. No husband or wife perfectly loves the other all of the time. We are sinful, selfish creatures. No matter how honorable our intentions are nor how hard we try, we inevitably serve ourselves in the end. For this reason, it is very important to remind ourselves and each other that we are forgiven in Christ Jesus. We can boldly confess our transgressions to God, for He promises to forgive us in Jesus' name.[2] We can also boldly confess our sins to each other, extending grace and forgiveness to our spouse because Christ first loves and forgives us.[3]

We all make mistakes and say hurtful things. None of us can stand blameless before the other. Thankfully, you know the blessed freedom that comes from being washed of your sins by the blood of the Lamb. With the help of the Holy Spirit, you can extend the same freedom of forgiveness to your spouse. It is this blessed freedom which can restore and heal your marriage, reconciling you to your husband and keeping you living as one flesh, in sickness and in health, so long as you both shall live.

---

2. Psalm 32:5; Psalm 130:3-4; Isaiah 1:18; John 14:13-14
3. Matthew 6:12; Matthew 18:21-22; Ephesians 4:32

## Reading

If you, O LORD, should mark iniquities,
    O Lord, who could stand?
But with you there is forgiveness,
    that you may be feared.
I wait for the LORD, my soul waits,
    and in his word I hope;
my soul waits for the Lord more than watchmen for the morning,
    more than watchmen for the morning.
O Israel, hope in the LORD!
    For with the LORD there is steadfast love,
    and with him is plentiful redemption.
And he will redeem Israel from all his iniquities. *Psalm 130:3-8*

## Collect

Let us pray … Heavenly Father, You created and instituted marriage to resolve mankind's alone-ness. Even now, after the Fall, You still bless this union. Send Your Holy Spirit to convict us to repentance when we sin against our spouse and move us to seek forgiveness from them and You. Direct all marriages to the cross. Remind us that we share in a perfect relationship with You through Jesus. Grant us thankful hearts for the blessing of a spouse, and beckon us to receive together Your gifts of forgiveness, life, and salvation through Your means of grace. In Jesus' Holy name. Amen.

## Hymn

We deserve but grief and shame,
    Yet, His words, rich grace revealing,
Pardon, peace, and life proclaim;
    Here our ills have perfect healing.
Firmly in these words believe:
    Jesus sinners doth receive.[4]

---

4. Erdmann Neumeister, "Jesus Sinners Doth Receive," tr. *The Lutheran Hymnal,* 1941 (*Lutheran Service Book,* 609), stanza 2.

# Chapter 12

# What If God Says No?

Would God, the great Creator of all life and the generous Giver of all good gifts, actually say no to our earnest pleas for a child? We know that God's revealed will for us in His Word is that we be receivers of His blessing of children.[1] Here we are, Lord! We are willing. We are ready. We are waiting. Yet, here we are today, still empty-handed, with no evidence that God intends to change our circumstances tomorrow.

Anna, for years, has been living in hope of what tomorrow might bring. Every night before going to bed, Anna pulls out a pad of paper and carefully writes down the things she needs to do the next day to accomplish her goals. Over the years, Anna's lists have changed: things to do to get pregnant; things to do to increase fertility; things to do to prepare for adoption; things to do to become certified by the state as a foster parent. Year after year, Anna has diligently applied herself to her lists in hope of becoming a parent, and, year after year, God has closed doors faster than Anna can make new lists.

The past year-and-a-half was particularly painful. Last Christmas, Anna and her husband Jeff were sought out by a local church and asked to open their hearts and home to a fatherless baby boy only to be told in the end that they were not qualified to adopt him. Last Spring, Jeff asked his employer to transfer him and his wife to

---

1. Psalm 127:3

a location where they could better afford to adopt a child, and, instead, his company moved them to a metropolitan area where local adoption costs exceeded twenty thousand dollars per child. Anna and Jeff spent the following summer working to fulfill the requirements for foster parent certification only to find out that the state would require them to reward foster children for such behaviors as masturbation, help and aid young girls seeking abortion, treat homosexuality as normal and healthy behavior, and tolerate the worshipping of false gods in their own home. Unable to agree to such things, Anna and Jeff let go of the last lifeline to which they were clinging, the one they hoped would pull them out of the sea of barrenness. Anna and Jeff had never considered the fact that God might say no to their plea for children, but life's circumstances certainly seemed to be delivering big, fat noes from every angle.

And, then, Anna became pregnant only to miscarry the same month.

It was all too much. Anna began to wonder if Satan and his minions would succeed in breaking her. She began to suffer from tension headaches and pains in her stomach caused by the ball of stress she swallowed every morning. She stayed in bed until the late morning hours and stopped answering her phone. She even lost her voice from the strain of crying hour after hour. Anna began to slide down the slippery slope of despair as a single, horrid truth sat heavy in her heart: "God may never give me a child."

Anna was no fool. She had been well catechized. She knew that God had not forgotten her. She knew that He couldn't. God's Word told her that she was adopted as His own child in her baptism.[2] Yet, even though Anna was His, she could not help feeling like her Heavenly Father was distant and removed, sitting on His throne in heaven, looking down in sorrow and pity as His own child became a chew toy in Beelzebub's mouth. Anna could almost feel Satan sinking his teeth into her neck, shaking and shaking her until she felt limp and lifeless. Satan whispered horrible ideas into Anna's ear in the darkness, and she began to doubt whether her petitions ever made it to the Divine Ear.

---

2. Galatians 3:26-4:7

Yet, God was not distant and removed. He had not left Anna alone to be senselessly battered and bruised in Sheol by the powers of darkness. There was not one tragedy that had come into Anna's life — or any of our lives, for that matter — without God's permission. As we learn from our brother Job, Satan can only deliver punches to Anna, you, and me which God allows. And, though Satan means it for evil, God means it all for our good.[3]

Does this comfort you? It comforts me. I am not a chew toy abandoned to the dogs of Hell! I am a child of God who suffers because God allows it, and He promises me in His Word that He will not give me more than I can handle.[4] He who raised Christ from the dead will lift me out of the muck and mire in His perfect time.[5] In the meantime, while I walk through the valley of the shadow of death, I will fear no evil. For God is with me. His rod and His staff, which can beat the pulp out of the devil at any moment He chooses, they really do comfort me. You and I have not been left alone to suffer. Instead, in our depravity and hunger, we are given second helpings of God's grace, mercy, and peace. We are weak, but He is strong. Take that, Devil!

We are broken in sin, and our brokenness will not be completely fixed until the Last Day. This is why our lives on earth seem to be in such contradiction with God's revealed will in His Word regarding procreation. Yes, God has commanded us to be fruitful and multiply. Yes, God wants to bless Christian marriages with the gift of children. Yet, our bodies still break, the world still reviles us, and we still live, like Anna, under the burden of childlessness. God has the power to heal us of our barrenness, but — honestly — it no longer really matters. God has already healed us from our sickness of sin at the font, and we are reconciled to Him for all of eternity. O, Resurrection Day, how we pine for thee! Come quickly, Lord Jesus!

You see, that is the gift God gives you and me in our childlessness. He makes the taste of resurrection even sweeter, so that we pine for it even more. That is why we can thank and praise Him, even when He tells us no. He frees us from the burden of living for

---

3. Genesis 50:20; Romans 8:28
4. 1 Corinthians 10:13
5. Psalm 31:15; Psalm 40:2

something that may or may not come tomorrow and, instead, helps us to live — no, thrive! — in the gift that is today by loving Him and serving our neighbor. We can throw away the lists and personal agendas of what we want to have happen, and, instead, respond to life's circumstances with faith in God Almighty who loves us completely in Jesus and promises to work all things for our good. We can speak aloud a hearty, "Amen!" at the end of the Lord's Prayer, trusting that when we pray the petition, "Thy will be done," it is indeed done. For, God promises to give ear to the petitions of His children, and we can rest in the assurance that He hears and answers our prayers.[6] Sometimes, we are even so blessed as Anna as to receive a "no."

Anna is just fine today, by the way, though she no longer puts so much hope in waiting for what God *might* give her. She grew weary of sacrificing all of her todays at the altar of her tomorrows. Instead, she takes great joy in the simple, comforting gift that God has brought her safely to another day in which she can live out her baptismal life in Christ. She still asks God to give her the gift of children, but she is not putting the rest of her life's vocations — wife, sister, daughter, friend — on hold until then. And, the only list she is making these days is for the groceries.

## Reading

Though I walk in the midst of trouble,
    you preserve my life;
You stretch out your hand against the wrath of my enemies,
    and your right hand delivers me.
The LORD will fulfill his purpose for me;
    your steadfast love, O LORD, endures forever.
Do not forsake the work of your hands. *Psalm 138:7-8*

---

6. Psalm 40:1

## Collect

Let us pray ... Heavenly Father, hear our pleas. When You return our works and desires with a "no," give us the peace to submit to Your will. Lead us not into temptation or despair. Stir up in us the understanding that Satan has no power over us though we live amongst his shadows. You promise to comfort us, so as we endure rejection, anxiety, and lost opportunity, bestow on us the fortitude to stand on Your Word. We look to You to send Your Holy Spirit to fill our wanting cups. Give us the strength to say, "Thy will be done," in all things temporal and eternal and to receive Christ's atonement at the cross as the answer to both. Kyrie eleison. Lord, have mercy. Amen.

## Hymn

What God ordains is always good:
    This truth remains unshaken.
Though sorrow, need, or death be mine,
    I shall not be forsaken.
        I fear no harm,
        For with His arm
He shall embrace and shield me;
    So to my God I yield me.[7]

---

7. Samuel Rodigast, "What God Ordains Is Always Good," tr. *The Lutheran 'ymnal*, 1941 (*Lutheran Service Book*, 760), stanza 6.

# Chapter 13

# Is It Okay for Me *Not* to Be a Mother?

Robin looked at me over her coffee one afternoon and confessed, "I feel worse for Bill than for myself. I see the way he interacts with other peoples' children. He is so tender with them. Bill tells me that he loves that it is just the two of us, but I feel so guilty."

Robin and Bill married later in life. They both had nurtured hopes of getting pregnant in the early years of their marriage, but nothing ever came of it. Now that Robin was in her mid-forties, neither of them expected to ever have any children.

"Why do you feel guilty?" I asked.

Robin shrugged her shoulders. "I don't know. I guess it is because I am okay with not being a mother. I mean, I used to be sad about it, but now I feel fine. Does that make me strange? Am I selfish?" Robin leaned forward over her coffee. "Do you think it is okay for me *not* to be a mother?"

I can understand Robin's confusion. There is no denying the fact that one of the purposes of marriage is procreation. God tells us in His Word that He loves life and wants children to be the blessed fruit of the one-flesh union between spouses.[1] It is not surprising, then, that a barren woman may feel guilty when her womb does not produce such God-pleasing fruit. That is why it is so important for us to remember that having children is not a law of God for us to keep but a heritage from Him for us to receive. It is not that we are

---

1. John 3:16; Psalm 127:3

unwilling to have children but that we are unable to have children. We do not need to fret that we are somehow guilty of not keeping the law if we, in our barrenness, are childless. Barrenness, after all, is not a sin.

I remember feeling particularly convicted in church one Sunday when my pastor preached a sermon on the Apostle Paul's first letter to Timothy: "[A woman] will be saved through childbearing."[2] The knife of the law cut through my chest as I sat in the pew, and my heart turned cold. How am I to be saved? I lowered my eyes in shame, certain that everyone else in the church was accusing me by name in their hearts.

I cried to my husband that afternoon. "What hope is there for a childless woman like me? How am I to be saved?"

My husband rushed in with the blessed, sweet Gospel that perfectly answers such a brutal law. "You *are* saved through childbearing, just not your own. Mary bore the Child that brings your salvation. Your hope — all of our hope — is in Jesus." Amen!

Just as our salvation is no less valid because our wombs are barren, our marriages are no less valid because they do not produce any children. God intended marriage for the mutual companionship, help, and support of every man and wife, and those are things we can still do for and enjoy in each other in spite of our barrenness. If God wills for us not to have children in our marriage, then we should simply rest in His will and, to the best that we can, rejoice. Sometimes, that may even mean rejoicing when others in the church think we should be grieving.

Robin laughed nervously. "Did you know that some women still come up to me after church to tell me they are praying for me to have a child? I am forty-six years old! Do these women think I am married to Abraham or something?"

Robin tried to make light of the situation, but I could see the pain that still resonated in her eyes. I watched as she squeezed her coffee cup tightly between both hands.

"I know they mean well," Robin said, "but it makes me feel guilty for being happy. I seriously think those women half expect me to

---

2. 1 Timothy 2:15, ESV

spend all of my days wearing black, mourning for what might have been." She sighed. "What is wrong with being content with the life God has given me?"

Nothing. Nothing at all. It is good and healthy to be content with the will of God. All the same, however, we must be careful not to let our contentedness grow into apathy. There is a fine line between being truly content in barrenness and being closed-hearted to the idea of being parents. Straddling this line is a cross that each barren couple must daily bear, for God instructs all husbands and wives to be open to His gift of children and welcome them in marriage, even when it means possibly suffering the pain of being denied such a gift month after month.

The emotional fatigue of continuing to want something you may never have is draining on any marriage. At some point, every one of us is tempted to adopt measures that may protect ourselves from continual disappointment and pain. For example, some couples, after years of trying to get pregnant with no success, find themselves avoiding sexual intimacy during the fertile days of each month. It may not even be a conscious decision on their part, but the couple falls into a pattern of abstaining in order to avoid the pain of crushed hopes at the end of each cycle. We must guard ourselves from such patterns of behavior that attempt to "play God" in our own lives and in the lives of each other. In truth, such measures do not really bring true comfort in the end but, instead, sabotage the already precarious balance of intimacy and trust in the one-flesh union between a barren couple.

Explore the lighter side of barrenness. (*Yes, you read that correctly.*) Recognize that your family life is going to look and feel very different from that of other married couples who have children. Rather than coveting that which you have not been given, celebrate that which you have. You and your husband enjoy a special freedom of schedule and resources that many parents would trade their minivan for in a heartbeat. Spend some of that money you have saved on a second honeymoon. Go out for breakfast every Tuesday morning and take dancing lessons on Thursday nights. Make it your goal this year to find the best bed and breakfast in the county. Take each other on impromptu, late-night coffee shop dates and stay up late talking about your days. Linger in bed on Saturday mornings as long as you want. Delight in each other and frequently practice your conjugal rights, enjoying each other for each other's sake.

Whatever you decide to do, remember that — barren or not — God still commands you to love and serve your neighbor. Barrenness is not some kind of divine permission for each of us to live a life of leisure void of any social responsibility. Quite the opposite, barrenness is divine permission for us to live a life in service of other parents and their children. In some cases, it may even mean providing primary care for children who have no homes.

Robin and Bill may already be past the age of child-bearing, but there are still many ways in which they can serve as parents in the church. They can befriend a younger couple who lives far away from their own family, acting as surrogate grandparents to the younger couple's children. They can sit in the same pew as a single mother, offering extra hands to help wrangle her kids during the service. They can purchase presents every Christmas for children in the congregation whose families are undergoing hard times. They can even serve as foster parents to children who have no homes of their own. The list of ways Bill and Robin can parent others in the church is endless.

Robin's eyes twinkled at me over her cup. "Bill and I have an idea." She took an envelope out of her purse and slid it across the table to me. "Open it."

I looked at her curiously.

"Go on," she laughed. "Don't take forever!"

I slid my finger along the flap and broke the seal. Reaching into the envelope, I pulled out a small, single piece of paper. It was a check with my husband's name written on it. I gasped when I saw the amount. "What is — ?"

"Now, don't make a scene!" Robin said. "Bill and I talked it over and we are going to mail you two a check like this every month."

I shook my head. "Robin, there is no way we can — "

"I don't want to hear it," Robin interrupted, her mouth twitching with delight. "We are so proud of Michael for entering the seminary, and we know how much it costs. These next four years are not going to be a cakewalk for either of you." She looked me squarely in the eye. "This is something Bill and I can do for both of you. This is something we *want* to do."

Tears flooded my eyes and spilled over onto my cheeks. "I don't know what to say."

"Don't say anything." Robin unceremoniously took the check out of my hand, put it back in the envelope, and stuffed it in my purse. "There. It's done."

Robin signaled for the waitress to bring the bill. When she turned back to me, her face was light and free of care. "If you think about it, Bill and I are really giving a gift to God, not to you." Robin winked and scooted out of the booth. "So, don't even think about wasting the postage to send us thank-you cards every month!"

As I followed Robin out the door of the restaurant, I pondered the sudden change in her countenance. What had happened in the last few minutes to chase the tension and fear from her eyes? What had replaced her doubt and pain with joy and delight? As I fumbled for my keys in my purse, my fingers brushed against the answer.

God granted Robin sweet relief from her barrenness — not by giving her the gift of children — but by giving her the means by which to mother me. In tending to the suffering of her neighbor, Robin found respite from her own.

## Reading

How precious is your steadfast love, O God!
    The children of mankind take refuge in the shadow of your wings.
They feast on the abundance of your house,
    and you give them drink from the river of your delights.
For with you is the fountain of life;
    in your light do we see light. *Psalm 36:7-9*

## Collect

Let us pray . . . Heavenly Father, Your work and blessings manifest themselves in our lives through means. Sometimes we try to seek, force, and manipulate people and things to fit our own selfish desires and misgivings about Your will. Please lead us not into temptation but deliver us from evil. Reassure us that You promise to shelter us in all storms, wants, and pain. Only in Your Son do we find true contentment. Thank You for all Your gifts. May we realize the eternal joy and peace we have received from Christ in our baptism and gladly share them with our neighbors. Amen.

## Hymn

Lord of glory, You have bought us
    With Your lifeblood as the price,
Never grudging for the lost ones
    That tremendous sacrifice.
Give us faith to trust You boldly,
    Hope, to stay our souls on You;
But, oh, best of all Your graces,
    With Your love our love renew.[3]

---

3. Eliza S. Alderson, "Lord of Glory, You Have Bought Us" (*Lutheran Service Book*, 851), stanza 4.

# Chapter 14

## He Remembers the Barren

When Noah was floating over the flooded earth in a wooden ark, God remembered him. God caused a wind to blow so that the waters would subside. He closed the fountains of the deep and the windows of heaven, restraining the rains so that the water would recede. God had mercy on Noah, his family, and all the beasts in the ark, bringing them safely onto dry land.

When the Israelites were held in slavery, God remembered them. He outstretched His arm and performed great acts of judgment on the Egyptians. He sent Moses to lead the Israelites out of the land of Egypt and across the great desert. God was favorable to the Israelites, freeing them from their burdens and bringing them to the land He swore to give to Abraham, Isaac, and Jacob.

When Hannah wept bitterly, God remembered her. He looked upon her affliction and listened to her prayer. He opened her womb that she might conceive and bear a son, giving her a child which would both silence her rival and grow up to speak the Word of the Lord to all of Israel. God knew Hannah as His own servant and granted her petition for the good of all of His children.

In the Hebrew language, the word "remember" is a relationship word. When God remembers someone in the Old Testament, He loves them, has mercy on them, is favorable to them, and, simply put, knows them. God still remembers His people today. He remembers *you*. He loves you, has mercy on you, and is favorable to

95

you in Christ Jesus. He has a relationship with you because of what Christ did for you on the cross. You put on Christ in your baptism, and now God knows you as His child and heir.[1] Your name is written in the Book of Life,[2] and you are remembered by Him unto life everlasting.

You may feel forgotten. You may think that God has passed over you in favor of others, but that is not true. God does not ignore your pain and suffering, nor does He wish for you to be childless. Your barrenness is not a curse from Him but a terrible consequence of living in a fallen world. It is evidence, not of God's rejection, but of man's sinfulness.

God is anything but oblivious to your pain. He suffers with you, going down into the depths of Sheol to pull you out with His own, pierced hands. He knows you in your baptism and loves you as His own, forgiving your sins and strengthening your faith through the hearing of His Word and the partaking of His Holy Supper. God may not open your womb as He did Hannah's, but He, in His wisdom, still remembers you every day by providing all that you need to support this body and life.

Look at how God remembers Robin, Katherine, and Carol in their barrenness. Robin and Bill, blessed with many good gifts in their marriage, are able to share those good gifts with others, serving as parents to the body of Christ. Katherine and Paul, blessed with the freedom to make family decisions which only directly affect each other, are both able to return to school for full-time graduate work in their respective fields, enjoying what they call their second "academic honeymoon." Carol and her husband, blessed with financial stability after years of earning two incomes, recently took a trip to Greece to retrace the steps of the Apostle Paul and are planning a hiking trip along the Appalachian Trail for this summer.

God remembers Beth, Sara, and Anna in different ways, as well. Beth started a knitting group that meets every Wednesday night in her church's parish hall. Together, she and the other women knit scarves and blankets for the men and women who serve in the mili-

---

1. Galatians 3:27-4:7
2. Philippians 4:3; Revelation 21:27

tary. Remembering the suffering and needs of others has helped her to reflect and meditate on just how much God remembers her own.

Sara no longer chases after fertility fads these days. Much to the bewilderment of all of her doctors and nutritionists, Sara and her husband got pregnant last Easter. No one is really certain which herbal cocktail did the trick, but Sara and her husband are certain of one thing: their child is a gift from God, a precious heritage from Him. They know with assurance that God remembers them.

Anna is living out her baptismal life to the fullest. She no longer sees her barrenness as a burden but as a gift. She has stopped expecting God to heal her broken body today, and, instead, thanks Him for His promise to make all things new on the Last Day. She rejoices in the very thing that makes her pine for the second advent of her Lord.

God remembers me, too. He still has not made me a mother of my own child, but He has made me a daughter, sister, wife, friend, teacher, aunt, godmother, and even a writer. I get to share in the suffering of my barren sisters in Christ, and, in return, celebrate the joy and peace they experience in Christ's love. I still ask that the Lord will remove this cup of barrenness from me, but, just as Jesus showed me in the Garden of Gethsemane, I can — through His strength — trust in the Father's perfect will. There is no denying that good things have come to all of us through Christ's own suffering on the cross, and I am comforted knowing that more good things can come to me from my own suffering.

God has not forgotten you. He knows you and loves you as His own. He sustains and preserves you in Him, strengthening your faith in the midst of suffering. Just as God saved Noah in the ark, so He saves you through the waters of Holy Baptism. Just as God led the Israelites out of the bondage of slavery, so He leads you safely from the bondage of sin into the Promised Land. Just as God opened Hannah's womb that she might bear a son, so He opens your barren heart that you might bear good fruit in service to your neighbor. Just as God has given good gifts to Robin, Katherine, Carol, Beth, Sara, Anna, me, and all of your barren sisters in Christ, so He gives good gifts to you. God remembers you, dear sister, and He will bless you and keep you, make His face to shine upon you and be gracious unto you, lift up His countenance upon you, and give you peace — all because you are His in Christ Jesus. Thanks be to God!

## Reading

O LORD my God, I cried to you for help
and you have healed me.
O LORD, you have brought up my soul from Sheol;
you restored me to life from among those who go down to the pit.
Sing praises to the LORD, O you his saints,
and give thanks to his holy name.
For his anger is but for a moment,
and his favor is for a lifetime.
Weeping may tarry for the night,
but joy comes with the morning.
You have turned for me my mourning into dancing;
you have loosed my sackcloth
and clothed me with gladness,
that my glory may sing your praise and not be silent.
O LORD my God, I will give thanks to you forever!
*Psalm 30:2-5, 11-12*

## Collect

Let us pray ... Heavenly Father, You remember us even when we so often forget about You. Teach us, we pray, to understand that Your remembrance is an eternal relationship forged for us through Jesus at the cross. Help us to faithfully receive Your Son, our Savior. Direct our hearts and minds to Your Word and Your Holy Supper, where Christ has promised to be. Your Word is truth, Your promises never fail, and you enrich our lives through this veil of tears. Help us to remember our baptism, our home away from home, till we see you face to face in heaven. In Jesus' name we pray. Amen.

## Hymn

What God ordains is always good:
　　He is my friend and Father;
He suffers naught to do me harm
　　Though many storms may gather.
　　　　Now I may know
　　　　Both joy and woe;
Someday I shall see clearly
　　That He has loved me dearly.[3]

---

3. Samuel Rodigast, "What God Ordains Is Always Good," tr. *The Lutheran ymnal*, 1941 (Lutheran Service Book, 760), stanza 4.

# A Note from the Author

The women you read about in this book are real, though their names and circumstances have been altered to protect individual privacy. It is my hope and intent, as well as that of every woman who generously shared her story for this publication, that these life experiences be a source of empathy and comfort to all of you in your suffering.

It is also my hope and intent that this conversation about barrenness not end here. In this life, God has called and ordained men to be pastors to stand before us in the stead of Christ. Please, go to your shepherd and let him take care of you. Confess to him your thoughts, your sufferings, your burdens, and your sins. Let him minister to you, speak God's Word to you, absolve you, and pray for you. He is there to help shoulder your burdens, and he wants to do just that.

In the inevitable circumstance that your pastor disappoints you, please forgive him. Pray for him. Be patient with him. Listen to him. Speak to him in kindness and love. He is, after all, another man for whom Christ died, and he will learn from you what it is like to be a barren woman.

Thank you for listening. It has helped me through the darkest of days to talk with you, to know that we are one in the body of Christ. Should you ever need someone to listen, it would be my privilege to return the favor.

HeRemembersTheBarren.com

KatieSchuermann.com

# Appendix I

# Why Did It Have to Be My Baby?

Carol leaned against the doorbell, balancing a pan of lasagna in one hand and a small, paper bag in the other. The dark, quiet house before her appeared to be sleeping, but Carol knew better. The porch light flickered on and a scruffy-chinned man opened the door.

"I brought you some lasagna, Mark," Carol said, holding out the pan. "I thought you and Gina might need something to eat for supper tonight."

Mark took the pan and stared at it, unseeing. "Thank you, Carol. I honestly had forgotten about supper."

Carol held up the paper bag. "I also brought a little something for Gina. Do you think she would like some company? I can leave it with you if you think she would rather be alone."

"No, I think it would be nice for her to see you." Mark stepped aside to let Carol into the house. "Gina is upstairs in the nursery. I'll just put this lasagna in the oven while you two talk."

Carol found Gina sitting in a rocking chair, mindlessly fingering the corded edge of a pillow on her lap. Carol sat down on a stool next to the rocking chair and set the paper bag at her feet. Neither woman said anything for a few moments.

"Are you in any pain?" Carol finally asked.

Gina continued fingering the pillow. "I can't feel a thing." Suddenly, Gina clutched the pillow to her stomach, squeezing her eyes shut against the world. Her face twisted to fight back the tears. "My baby is dead, and I can't feel a thing," she sobbed.

Carol reached out and grabbed her friend's knee. Her voice was calm and steady. "What did the ultrasound technician say this morning?"

Gina took in a shaky breath. "She said that the baby died at eight weeks. That was five weeks ago. How can my baby have died five weeks ago and I not have known it?"

"What are you going to do?" Carol asked.

Gina shook her head from side to side. "I don't know. The technician said that we can either remove the baby or wait for my body to miscarry it naturally."

"What does Mark think?"

"Mark thinks we should go ahead and have a D&C tomorrow, but I am scared. What if the baby isn't really dead? What if the technician is wrong?" Gina's voice broke. She wept into the pillow, hiding her face.

Carol held onto her friend's knee for dear life. "I am so sorry, Gina."

"It was awful," Gina continued in a muffled voice. "After the ultrasound, Mark and I had to walk back through the lobby. All of the women sitting there looked so happy. I hated every one of them." Gina looked up. "Why did it have to be my baby? Why couldn't it have been one of theirs, instead?"

Carol sat in silence, waiting.

"I prayed every day for the health of this child. Why did God let my baby die?" Gina asked, unrelenting. Her eyes were red and swollen.

Carol still waited.

"I trusted God to protect my baby, and He broke His promise to me."

Carol finally opened her mouth to speak. "God never breaks His promises to you." She looked into her friend's eyes with compassion. "It is unfair and cruel that you lost your baby, but God never promised health and happiness for you or your child. His promise to us are for forgiveness and salvation, and those He gives to us in abundance through Jesus."

Gina shook her head. " But, I want my baby here with me."

"I want my baby here with me, too," Carol said.

Gina stared at Carol. The room was very still. Carol spoke softly, carefully holding Gina's gaze. "David and I lost a child two years before we met you and Mark. Our baby girl died in my womb. She would be four years old if she were alive today."

Gina sat in bewildered silence. She opened her mouth as if to say something, but no words came out. Instead, she tentatively reached out to take Carol's hand. The two women sat in silence together, each lost in her own thoughts. When Gina spoke, her voice was dull. "I don't want to live if my baby is dead."

"I know," Carol said quietly.

"How did you get through it?" Gina asked.

"I am still getting through it," Carol said. "Every time I see a child in church or at the grocery store, my heart hurts. Every day is a reminder of the fact that my child is not with me."

"Do you think your baby is in heaven?" Gina whispered.

Carol sat still for a moment. She chose her next words very carefully. "Scripture tells me that God knit my daughter together in my womb. I know that she was fearfully and wonderfully made by Him. God is both her Creator and Savior, just as He is mine. Whether we die in the womb or out of it, we all rest in the mercy and grace of Christ. That is my comfort."

"Is my baby in heaven?" Gina barely breathed.

Carol squeezed Gina's hand tightly. "Think of how John the Baptist leapt in Elizabeth's womb at the sound of the mother of his Lord! We know that babies in the womb can have faith." Carol looked her friend squarely in the face. "You also just told me that you have been praying for your child, and Jesus promises that He hears our prayers. Have faith in His promises, Gina. Trust that God's grace extends even to your child."

"Why did He take my baby?" Gina asked.

"It was never *your* baby," Carol said gently. "Children are a gift from the Lord. We are simply stewards of His good gifts to us. 'The Lord giveth, and the Lord taketh away; blessed be the name of the Lord.'"

"Why couldn't He have taken me, instead?" Fresh tears splashed onto Gina's shirt.

"Death is certain for all of us. It is only the timing that is uncertain." Carol leaned forward. "It is not for you or me to decide when each of us will fall asleep in Jesus."

"Did I do something wrong?" Gina cried.

Carol's voice was firm. "Your baby didn't die because of you. Your baby died because this world is cursed. Sin messed it up, and now we all have been given the death sentence. The wages of sin for *every* person is death, even for our babies." Carol's eyes were on fire. "Praise God for Jesus! Praise God He sacrificed His one and only Son on the cross to pay our debt for us! In Jesus, we have hope. In Jesus, we look forward to eternal life in heaven where death no longer threatens us."

Gina silently hugged the pillow to her chest.

"God loves you and your baby so much that He gave up His Son, so that all who believe in Him can live eternally with Him." Carol leaned back. "You see, Gina, God knows what it is like to lose a child."

Gina looked up at Carol, her lips trembling. "I never even got to meet my baby."

Carol reached down into the paper bag on the floor and pulled out a small, white lamb. A purple ribbon was tied around its neck. She handed it to Gina. "I knitted this for you today."

Gina took the lamb in her hands and fingered the soft yarn.

"I never got to hold my baby, either," Carol explained. "After my miscarriage, I kept wishing I had something physical and tangible to hold, something that would help me remember her. I knitted you this lamb, so that you would have something to hold tomorrow and every day after that."

Tears slid down Gina's face.

Carol slowly stood up. "Gina, would you let me call Pastor Schmidt for you? I know that he would want to know how you are suffering. He would want to be here with you and Mark tonight."

Gina sat in silence, unmoved.

"God has not left you here to endure the sorrows of this day alone," Carol said. "Pastor Schmidt is your shepherd. Christ has put him here in His stead to care for you. May I please call him for you?"

Gina stared at the lamb for a few moments and then nodded her head. Carol could smell the lasagna cooking in the kitchen downstairs. She turned to walk towards the door.

"Carol," Gina suddenly called out, grabbing Carol's hand. Her eyes were panicked. "All I ever wanted was to be a mother."

Carol looked kindly into her friend's eyes. "You are still a mother. Today has not changed that." She gently tugged on Gina's hand. "Why don't you come downstairs with me, while I call Pastor Schmidt? Mark is making supper. It would be good to check on him. He has had a long day, too."

Gina stood up from the rocking chair to follow Carol. The pillow fell from her lap to the floor, forgotten. Gina was too busy cradling her little lamb to notice.

## Reading

Truly God is good to Israel,
    to those who are pure in heart.
But as for me, my feet had almost stumbled,
    my steps had nearly slipped.
For I was envious of the arrogant
    when I saw the prosperity of the wicked.
But when I thought how to understand this,
    it seemed to me a wearisome task,
until I went into the sanctuary of God;
    then I discerned their end.
When my soul was embittered,
    when I was pricked in heart,
I was brutish and ignorant;
    I was like a beast toward you.
Nevertheless, I am continually with you;
    you hold my right hand.
You guide me with your counsel,
    and afterward you will receive me to glory.

Whom have I in heaven but you?
>And there is nothing on earth that I desire besides you.
My flesh and my heart may fail,
>but God is the strength of my heart and my portion forever.
For behold, those who are far from you shall perish;
>you put an end to everyone who is unfaithful to you.
But for me it is good to be near God;
>I have made the Lord GOD my refuge,
>that I may tell of all your works. *Psalm 73:1-3, 16-17, 21-28*

## Collect

Let us pray . . . Heavenly Father, our hearts are heavy when we recall others' or our own experiences with death, especially the death of an unborn child. Before we can touch the flesh of this new life, it is gone, with only the remnants of personal unfulfilled wishes, hopes, and dreams left. Be with the mothers who must endure the physical and emotional hardships that this brings. Send Your holy angels to attend to them and their loved ones, as temptations to doubt Your good and gracious will may creep into their minds. Assure us all that death has no sting since You are not its Creator, and that You only pour out blessings of forgiveness, life, and salvation in Jesus Christ. Let this be a comfort to all, as we come to know that faith is not something we can do, but something we simply receive from You, even in the womb. In Jesus' name we pray. Amen.

## Hymn

Who so happy as I am,
Even now the Shepherd's lamb?
>And when my short life is ended,
>By His angel host attended,
He shall fold me to His breast,
There within His arms to rest.[1]

---

1. Henrietta L. von Hayn, "I Am Jesus' Little Lamb," tr. *The Lutheran Hymnal*, 1941 (*Lutheran Service Book*, 740), stanza 3.

# Appendix II

## Pilates and Cosmos
### by Dcs. Melissa A. DeGroot

For every story, there is a back story. My journey with Katie to the completion of *He Remembers the Barren* has been an incredible experience. But many of you know only the half of it: Katie's. But I have to tell the readers my perspective on how this whole book came into being. (Oh, and Katie . . . this is my story, and I'm sticking to it.)

It all started in the late spring of 2008 with an invitation to a pilates session at Katie's apartment. First, a little, important aside: I used to be a track coach and personal trainer. While pilates is beneficial, it is not my preferred workout. My personal exercise mantra is "if you're not crying for your momma by the end of it, is it really worth it?"

So thankfully, after the morning spent with three other wives squeezed across Katie's living room floor (laughing and bumbling through the DVD), I discovered that it wasn't Katie's preferred way to "get her sweat on," either. That very day we planned to continue working out together in the seminary gym and invited anyone else who wanted to experience an "exercise beating," to join us.

We had some takers, but most early mornings only Katie and I blazed the treadmills and pumped iron together. It was glorious . . . and brutal.

Working out has always been both physical and social for me, and this partnership proved to develop into a friendship I never expected. Like every other seminary wife, we had one major thing in common. We were married to men who were studying to become pastors. Our personal histories, adventures and mishaps about marriage and seminary life were discussed fully and freely over the bench press and squat rack that summer. And thankfully, they still are today.

We learned a lot about each other in between the 'oh-so-feminine' gym grunts. Katie learned I was a deaconess working in admissions at the seminary, but I discovered that she worked for a satellite university in Fort Wayne, and is a very talented vocalist. And now, as you might have noticed, a very talented writer.

One other common bond was we both didn't have children.

That last detail surfaced a few workouts later. I think I just came out and asked her about it. I don't recall my exact words or tone, but I could tell it was a sensitive subject. The topic later eased into our talks more naturally, and it wasn't long before I began to understand how much children, fertility, and barrenness were important issues to Katie.

In late July 2008, I had registered for a "Writing for the Church" workshop that was being held in St. Louis. So a few days before, I explained to Katie I'd be out of town that week and that we could pick up working out together when I returned. (I think I even gave her an exercise schedule to do while away!)

But in the final workout before my trip, she said, "You know, Melissa, I've been thinking an awful lot about this issue of barrenness. And now with you going to this workshop and you being a deaconess, I think you should write a spiritual care resource for barren women."

Ka-boom! The bomb had dropped.

I carefully absorbed the idea and went to St. Louis. While there, I wrote a preliminary outline for Katie's topic. The workshop was enlightening and helpful (it was, in fact, where I met an editor to jumpstart this book). But, steering my personal focus to tackle barrenness, and its spiritual care, was difficult. While I, too, didn't have children at the time, articulating the sufferings of a barren woman was not an area of particular passion, or expertise, for me.

I returned to Fort Wayne and reconvened with Katie. Like any other workout morning, we started warming up on the treadmill. She asked about the workshop, and I sputtered off the highlights. Then without hesitation, I looked over at her and plainly stated, "I think you need to write this book."

Then, the proverbial ball got rolling.

My husband and I moved to North Carolina in August 2008 for vicarage, and Katie remained in Fort Wayne with her husband for his last seminary year. But correspondence and visits between us never ceased.

Because I was telecommuting for the Admissions Department from our vicarage house in North Carolina, I needed to fly to Fort Wayne periodically. So, I would call up Katie, sometimes to meet in the mornings for a workout . . . but then usually later to eat at our Fort Wayne favorite, Cosmos, for breakfast, and to talk about whatever.

Months after our initial agreement that Katie should pioneer this project, a nod from an editor only increased our discussions on the book, along with many peoples' encouragements to see *He Remembers the Barren* in print. Katie finally disclosed to me her desire to move ahead with the project in May 2009. Like foraging to satisfy the pangs of hunger, Katie said she just couldn't wait any longer to write *He Remembers The Barren*. I was thrilled.

So it began. She wrote furiously, brain-dumping months of mental outlines and recorded interviews to their organized places on the computer pages, and into your hands now. I simply had the privilege of reading each chapter, and the small task of writing the collects. I can only credit myself for putting (shoving, perhaps) Katie's idea back onto her plate.

All of the theological expositions, hymn and Scripture choices, and interviews were researched and conducted by her. It was Katie who poured endless hours of original content — her heart and soul — into this book. So like the heir of a rich relative, I feel like I'm reaping the benefits of her good and gracious will to include me in in the ride. Maybe it was all the rancorous exercise that diluted her.

Either way, I am ever thankful for all the gifts God has given her and for her unconditional love and friendship to me.

With the help of God, the collects were written as composite reflections for each chapter. May this book be read to God's glory, for both personal uses and group discussions. I believe *He Remembers the Barren* resonates with all women, barren or not. It certainly did for me. May it be a soothing balm to each of your souls and a sobering conversation with our loving God.

Our Father's heavenly and earthly care for us all never ceases, whatever sufferings befall us. May we draw ever closer to Him, through Jesus Christ our Lord. Amen.

# Bibliography

"Ectopic Pregnancy & In Vitro Fertilization" with Dr. Kevin Voss, November 19, 2008. http://www.issuesetc.org/podcast/Show103111908H1S1.mp3

*The Holy Bible. English Standard Version.* Wheaton, Illinios: Crossway, 2001.

Luther, Martin. *Luther's Small Catechism with Explanation.* St. Louis: Concordia Publishing House, 1986.

*Lutheran Service Book.* St. Louis: Concordia Publishing House, 2006.

*Lutheran Service Book: Pastoral Care Companion.* St. Louis: Concordia Publishing House, 2007.

McGuire, Brent. Interview by author, tape recording. August 7, 2009.

Pless, John. Interview by author, tape recording. October 15, 2008.

Pulse, Jeffrey. Interview by author, tape recording. October 10, 2008.

Rasmussen, Adrienne. Interview by author, tape recording. October 31, 2009.

Wendorf, Kristine. Interview by author, tape recording. August 13, 2009.

# Thank you to:

... Michael, my beloved, for giving me the Gospel in the dark hours of the night. Thank you for loving me just as I am, in sickness and in health, in good times and in bad. Thank you for being my theological editor.

... Mom and Dad for teaching me that life is valuable and encouraging me to write about it.

... Melissa for coaching me on and off the treadmill. This book would not be but for you. You are one of God's good gifts to me in this life.

... Pastor Mark Taylor and Lutheran Legacy for being willing to publish a book that addresses barrenness and suffering, no matter how niche its market may be.

... Peggy Kuethe of Concordia Publishing House for giving me the green light to start this project and the confidence to see it through to its completion.

... Professor John T. Pless for teaching me that Christian ethics begin with language and for being an advocate for this book.

... Professor Jeffrey Pulse for pastoring me in my grief and for reminding me that the Old Testament really is all about Jesus.

. . . Pastor Kurt Ulmer for pointing out that lamentation is a fruit of faith in God.

. . . Pastor Brent McGuire for reminding me that I am remembered by God.

. . . Pastor William Cwirla for making sure that the words I write are the words I mean.

. . . Kristi Leckband and Kristen Gregory for being my sounding boards and faithful sources of encouragement.

. . . Adrienne Rasmussen and Rebecca Mayes for championing this book and giving hope to others who suffer.

. . . Jennifer, Crissy, and Lucy for teaching me how to be a mother to all children.

. . . Katherine for leading me to the hymnal for comfort.

. . . Julie for teaching me to see the silver lining.

. . . Kristine for reassuring me that God really is in control.

. . . Melissa, Alissa, Nora, Kristen, Jennifer, Kristi, Adrienne, Kristine, Julie, and so many other sisters in Christ who so generously share their stories with all of us.